JOHN URI LLOYD

JOHN URI LLOYD

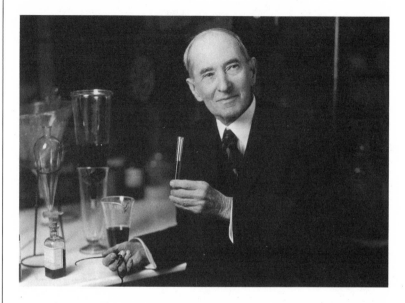

The Great American Eclectic

MICHAEL A. FLANNERY

SOUTHERN ILLINOIS UNIVERSITY PRESS

Carbondale and Edwardsville

Printed in the United States of America

01 00 99 98   4 3 2 1

Library of Congress Cataloging-in-Publication Data
Flannery, Michael A., 1953–
John Uri Lloyd : the great American eclectic / Michael A. Flannery.
p.   cm.
Includes bibliographical references and index.
1. Lloyd, John Uri, 1849–1936.   2. Medicine, Eclectic—Ohio—Cincinnati—
Biography.   3. Pharmacists—Ohio—Cincinnati—Biography.   I. Title.
RV76.L56F53   1998
615′.1′092—dc21
[B]
97-29242
CIP
ISBN 0-8093-2167-X (cloth : alk. paper)

Title page: John Uri Lloyd in his laboratory (ca. 1915).
Courtesy of the Lloyd Library and Museum, Cincinnati, Ohio.

The paper used in this publication meets the minimum requirements of
American National Standard for Imformation Sciences—Permanence of Paper
for Printed Library Materials, ANSI Z39.48–1984. ♾

for Alex

In my opinion biographical studies should be designed not so much to give individual records, as to use individual records as a string to which useful and interesting side studies are attached. Surely the string that I have followed has not been paralleled in American pharmacy, and it should not be lost.

—*John Uri Lloyd to Edward Kremers,*
May 21, 1920

Contents

Illustrations

Preface

Kremers and Urdang's History of Pharmacy, the leading textbook on the subject, has acknowledged John Uri Lloyd as "one of the greatest and most versatile pharmacists that America has had." Lloyd conducted pioneer research in fluidextracts, work recognized by his colleagues in the award of three Ebert Prizes for original research in pharmacy. His widely utilized book *The Chemistry of Medicines* (1st ed. 1881) was one of the first such texts published in America. Lloyd's professional leadership won him the presidency of the American Pharmaceutical Association in 1887–1888, and his work on elixirs helped lead the way to the first national formulary in 1888. Moreover, Lloyd's assistance with the U.S. government in implementing the Spanish-American War tax, his role in the introduction of important principles in chemistry to pharmacy, and his ventures into fiction all warrant the high praise bestowed upon this American pharmacist. Consequently, a book-length study of the life of such an important personage immediately suggests itself. Indeed his versatility allows us to see not only American pharmaceutical development but also key features in the emergence of modern chemistry, the growth of modern medicine and medical education, the retrenchment of medical sectarianism, and the decline and phoenixlike rebirth of interest in medicinal plants. Beyond science, however, Lloyd's literary endeavors, his founding of a major research library, and his work with the government provide us with a broader picture of American life from the Victorian age through the first decades of this century. Thus the life of John Uri Lloyd epitomizes what Barbara Tuchman, in *Practicing History*, considers the chief characteristic of all good biography: "useful because it encompasses the universal in the particular."

One would never have guessed his importance by his physical stature. He was short (only about five feet, four inches tall) and slight of build. Childhood asthma gave him a weak voice, so weak in fact that his public speeches were often read by someone else. Even throughout most of his adult life he was nursing some cough or cold, and persistent allergies stood between him and his love of animals. Later in life his poor hearing limited his social engagements. But Lloyd had a powerful presence. A longtime teacher of pharmacy and chemistry, he could gain the respect of even the most disruptive students through his sheer command of the subject matter. When he addressed large audiences, Lloyd's characteristic raised finger followed by the announcement "Listen!" caused crowds to hush.

Of course it was not always this way. Like many an antebellum lad, Lloyd rose up from rustic surroundings. Although born in upstate New York, he moved very early in life to Kentucky, and to his dying day considered the commonwealth his home state. His parents were teachers and knew how to encourage their boy's insatiable curiosity and practical skills at constructing homemade experiments. Their efforts yielded results, for these remained Lloyd's chief attributes throughout his life and the keys to his success.

A typical day in the prime of Lloyd's adult life illustrates his amazingly facile mind. He would rise early and have breakfast in his comfortable Norwood, Ohio, home with his wife, Emma, and their three children. He then proceeded to his pharmaceutical manufacturing plant at Court and Plum Streets in downtown Cincinnati, where he would meet his younger brothers, Nelson Ashley and Curtis Gates. Around 10 A.M. he walked across the street to teach chemistry and pharmacy at his beloved Eclectic Medical Institute (EMI), where he also interacted with the faculty and caught up on the latest news in the medical profession. Afternoons were spent attending to correspondence and his lab work at the Lloyd Brothers firm. Not infrequently, if he became immersed in a particularly intriguing problem, his experiments might continue well into the night; otherwise he was home in the evenings conjuring up another chapter in one of his Stringtown novels before turning in for the night. Lloyd's diversity can be seen in this twenty-four-hour summary: In a single day he assumed the roles of husband and father, businessman, teacher, colleague, professional confidant and consultant, chemist, researcher, and literary author. This is a lot of ground to cover for any man, but Lloyd reveled in it.

Lloyd's professional interests were largely shaped by his early associations with, and continued devotion to, eclecticism. Eclecticism can be briefly described as a nineteenth-century sectarian medical movement emerging out of Americans' dissatisfaction with the harsh heroic therapies characteristic of regular (also referred to as allopathic) practitioners. Distrustful of European ideas and institutions, eclectics promoted botanical remedies drawn primarily from America's fields and forests rather than the chemical and mineral concoctions that formed much of the allopath's armamentarium. Unlike some of their unschooled counterparts, eclectics ceaselessly promoted formal medical training through the establishment of their own educational institutions. The leading such school was Cincinnati's Eclectic Medical Institute, founded in 1845 by the sect's missionary apostle, Thomas Vaughan Morrow. As their name would imply, they refused to adhere to any single medical dogma but rather were, at least in principle, open to any idea if it seemed efficacious. For nearly one hundred years, the EMI formed the central hub of these catholic notions in the healing arts.

Despite the eclectics' openness to different ideas, they did have some distinct preferences: Their interests resided primarily in vegetable materia medica, which made phytopharmaceuticals their therapeutic hallmark. As the sole manufacturer of John Milton Scudder's Specific Medicines, John Uri Lloyd quickly became *the* central figure of American eclecticism. Through his medicinal plant investigations, Lloyd contributed not only to eclecticism but to pharmacy in general, and herein lies his claim to greatness. By devoting himself to creating new, better, and more standardized preparations for eclectics, he also contributed to pharmacy by enhancing his generation's understanding of medicinal plant constituents, phytochemistry, colloidal chemistry, and pharmaceutical manufacturing processes. He was one of leading pharmacists of his age at least in part *because* of his eclecticism.

Lloyd was also eclectic in the vernacular sense, actively engaging in very different activities, often concurrently. To escape from the cares of his profession, for example, Lloyd wrote fiction. The first of these efforts took the interesting and somewhat eccentric form of an inner-earth adventure titled *Etidorhpa*. Published in 1895, it has had a long and curious printing history and is still sought after as a cult classic by New Agers and science fiction enthusiasts. The remainder of his literary endeavors, however, were more conventional. Capitalizing on the immense popularity of regional fiction, Lloyd's local color tales of his boyhood home in northern Kentucky created a brief but noteworthy sensation among the reading public of his day.

Another activity demonstrating Lloyd's eclectic nature was his friendship with Grover Cleveland. Always an ardent Democrat, Lloyd's association with the former president gave him a certain amount of name recognition among men in Washington. Lloyd was, therefore, sometimes consulted on governmental affairs when issues touched on pharmaceutical manufacturing or research issues. His civic interests also involved him in local Cincinnati politics. He is perhaps the only pharmacist ever asked by reform-minded citizens to become mayor of a major American city.

Lloyd's career traversed a revolutionary transformation in the health care sciences as well as socioeconomic and cultural life in the United States. The medicine and pharmacy of Lloyd's youth was fundamentally different by the time of Lloyd's octogenarian years, and Lloyd's role in and response to those paradigmatic changes forms a significant part of this story. During his life the old-time "office pharmacy" practiced by individual physicians became increasingly rare as more college-trained pharmacists entered the field and assumed a more prominent role in compounding. This function too was gradually to become less prevalent as pharmacists became more involved in dispensing prefabricated dosage forms produced by a growing pharmaceutical industry. Those wanting to know more about the general development of the health care industry in the United States will also find Lloyd's life informative and illustrative, as he labored within this rapidly changing and highly volatile laissez-faire environment. His literary efforts may not have produced classics, but the endurance of his novel *Etidorhpa* and the record left by his Stringtown series are worth studying within the cultural context of Victorian America. In scientific research, literature, and business, Lloyd has a story to tell. It is a varied one of infighting, contention, and competition; but also one of enterprise, collaboration, and achievement.

I have attempted to render a picture of Lloyd "warts and all." Always concerned with his appearance and professional status, Lloyd himself might have preferred that I leave out a number of things in this book. Such an approach would, of course, serve no one. If this great American eclectic seems a bit blemished by my pen, he also appears more human. I hope that, rather than walking stiffly and stiltedly across the page, he will appear real, with his true accomplishments still intact. The degree to which I have achieved this goal is for the reader to judge.

That judgment, however, should be formed in the same manner as Lloyd's own eclectic activities—by a varied audience. In this regard I have attempted to cast a wide net, dealing with *all* aspects of Lloyd's diversity. Lloyd's profession naturally necessitates a certain amount of technical discussion regarding the nature of pharmaceutical practice during the last half of the nineteenth century, as well as fairly detailed and extended explanations of his work in colloidal chemistry. This book is designed to be read by the present generation of Lloyd's colleagues *and* by those who have merely been on the receiving end of the pre-scription counter. I have come to this study myself not as a pharmacist but as a librarian and a historian interested in conveying to the reading public a small part of this fascinating discipline's rich past.

Acknowledgments

I might never have written the biography of John Uri Lloyd had it not been for a chance meeting at the Lloyd Library some years ago with Dr. Alex Berman, a professor emeritus of history and historical studies in pharmacy at the University of Cincinnati. While I was working on a short article on Lloyd, a conversation ensued between myself and Dr. Berman, one of the library's longtime patrons. He encouraged my efforts and seemed to take a special interest in my historical interest in Lloyd. Obviously knowledgeable about American pharmacy, he was equally at home among French apothecaries. He was free with his knowledge, and I was eager to learn.

Since that time a number of changes have occurred. I am now director of the library founded by the subject of this biography, and the research that produced several journal articles has now grown into the present book. Alex Berman has been with me every step of the way in this project—consulting, consoling, advising, and correcting from beginning to end. If this study succeeds in its goal of objectively portraying one of American pharmacy's best and brightest, it is because of the time and expertise bestowed by this kindly scholar upon this novice to the field. I dedicate this book to Alex Berman—scholar, counselor, friend.

Additionally, special appreciation goes to the American Institute of the History of Pharmacy (AIHP) for the award of its 1995 Fischelis grant. Without the institute's support, the requisite travel, research, translating, and correspondence could not have been undertaken. I sincerely hope that this biography exemplifies the institute's high standards of excellence in the field. In particular, I would like to thank Gregory J. Higby, the director of the AIHP, for assisting in my use and access of the Kremers Reference Files and for permission to reproduce the photograph of Charles Rice in this book.

Appreciation is also extended to Dr. Thomas H. Appleton Jr. and the Kentucky Historical Society for permission to incorporate material from my article "The Local Color of John Uri Lloyd" (*Register* 91 [winter 1993]: 24–50), as part of chapter 8.

As in all projects of this kind, the metamorphosis from draft to manuscript to book did not occur in a vacuum. I was fortunate to have had the assistance of several readers who examined various permutations of this work with a critical eye and made numerous helpful comments and suggestions. They are: John S. Haller, Jr., a professor of history and medical humanities, Southern Illinois University at Carbondale; John Parascandola, a U.S. Public Health Service historian; and James A. Ramage, a professor of history, Northern Kentucky University. The reading of chapter 5 by Patrick Belcastro, a professor emeritus of pharmaceutics at Purdue University, was extremely helpful. While each scholar's generous contribution of time and expertise was indispensable, any errors or omissions remain solely my responsibility.

I also want to thank the staff of the Lloyd Library and Museum. In particular, appreciation goes to Betsy Kruthoffer, an assistant librarian, who contributed to the expeditious completion of this project; I found it possible to devote many hours researching this biography because I knew the day-to-day operations of the library were in excellent hands. Also, Mary Lee Schmidt assisted in assembling much of the photographic material in this biography and provided technical help in creating duplicate camera-ready illustrations when needed. Finally, Rose Marie Weckenmann organized the mass of photocopies, correspondence, translation transcripts, and other materials emanating from this study. Except for the photograph of Charles Rice mentioned above, all photographs herein are from the museum's collection.

No acknowledgment would be complete without recognizing Dona, my wife and best friend, who spent many evenings and weekends with her husband glued to his word processor.

JOHN URI LLOYD

I

Lloyd's Early Years,
1849–1863

The first words ever written about John Uri Lloyd can be found in a short notation by an obscure country doctor. The small notebook with the handwritten title "List of Births & Deaths for 1847 to 1851" by Dr. Joseph Hall Sr., West Bloomfield, New York, showed 1849 to be an especially fruitful year for the small village in the Genesee Valley. With the spring still young and less than two weeks since his last delivery, Hall made the following entry: "April 19, 1849. Nelson M. Lloyd, child born a son. West Bloomfield Ontario County, N.Y."[1] Thus began the life of John Uri Lloyd, who would become one of the most colorful and versatile pharmacists ever to grace the American scene.

He came from "good stock." On his father's side, his great-grandfather, John Lloyd, was part of a hearty line of Welshmen who ventured to the New World about 1770 seeking (like so many others) a better life.[2] Like much of the restless American populace, he did not linger on the coast. Along the banks of the Honeoye River in the still untamed section of west central New York, he established a tannery to support his wife, Susan Chadwick Lloyd, and their growing family. John wisely reasoned that a tanner would be needed in an area of tremendous growth. New York was selling land at giveaway prices, and by the late 1780s land commissioners had sold more than 5.5 million acres of the state's interior as land-hungry families poured into the region.[3] The eldest of the Lloyd's children, John Lloyd Jr. (born in 1773), married Sarah Devoe and enlarged the Lloyds of western New York by twelve. Their eldest child became the industrious John Lloyd III, who would marry Orpha Gates

Lloyd. They christened their second child (born on June 27, 1821) Nelson Marvin. Determined to give their son all the advantages that they could afford, Nelson's parents sent him to Lima Seminary, where he acquired the skills of teaching and civil engineering. While teaching in Lima, New York, he married his teaching assistant Sophia Webster, on September 6, 1847.

John Uri Lloyd's maternal lineage was even more impressive. Sophia could trace her American heritage back to the Massachusetts Bay Colony when John Webster settled there in the 1630s.[4] Elijah Webster, John Uri Lloyd's great-grandfather, was originally from Litchfield, Connecticut, but at the age of thirty-three he brought his wife, Lois Coe Webster, and their growing family to western New York on the Mohawk River. The Websters of Connecticut were part of a veritable sea of New Englanders pouring into western New York. It was a race for land the sheer frenzy of which was demonstrated spectacularly in one three-day period in February of 1795 when twelve hundred sleighs passed through Albany headed for the rich bottomlands of the Genesee Valley.[5] Elijah and Lois Webster had preceded this wintry rush less than a year earlier. Despite Elijah's death shortly after his arrival in the western country, the five children survived through the perseverance of their mother and some kindly, prosperous uncles. One of these children was John Uri Lloyd's grandfather, Uri Webster, who at the age of twenty-nine married Mercy Ashley on January 6, 1812, and became a successful "machinist," whose business it was "to go about the country to erect cotton factories and get them into running order. Then he would take stock in the factory for his pay."[6] The income from these ventures was enough to make a comfortable living and send Uri and Mercy's bright and promising daughter Sophia to the school where she would meet her husband.

Thus, in an age when advanced study of any kind was a rarity reserved for the few who could afford it, John Uri Lloyd was born to talented and comparatively well educated parents: a father who was "gifted in mathematics" and a mother who possessed an "educational and literary mind."[7] Nelson Marvin Lloyd worked with several surveying parties constructing the New York Central Railroad and the Erie Canal aqueduct at Rochester while Sophia taught school in several towns in the area. In addition, Nelson became the principal of the Acad-

emy of West Bloomfield, where he was remembered by former pupils
"with a great deal of affection."[8]

When an opportunity to be a part of the ambitious project to sur- Lloyd's
vey a route for a rail line between Covington and Louisville in Ken- *Early Years,*
tucky presented itself in 1853, Nelson, like his father before him, struck *1849–1863*
out for the land of promise. It was a young and sturdy family that Nelson brought with him. His wife was used to the rigors of motherhood,
little "Johnny" was now four, and he had a two-year-old brother, Nelson
Ashley. They moved into a comfortable two-story brick home in
Burlington, Kentucky, the county seat and oldest incorporated town of
Boone County. Prospects in the Bluegrass State looked bright.

The area was even more rustic than the environs they had left. Aside
from some minor river trade (the bulk of which passed on to Cincinnati), Boone County could claim barely eleven thousand souls in 1850.
Although situated between two boom towns (Covington, a few miles
to the east, and Louisville, about eighty miles to the west), the county
itself showed few signs of growth, and it would take another century
before its population topped a mere thirteen thousand.[9] These were pre-
dominantly simple, hardworking tobacco farmers whose pastoral habits
and colorful speech offered a stark contrast to Cincinnati, the sophisticated Queen City just a few miles upstream. These people became an
intimate circle of friends and acquaintances for young Johnny Lloyd as
he was growing up, and as an adult he immortalized them in a series of
nostalgic local color stories to be discussed later. As the author of those
stories, Lloyd mused in third person that the people he described are
"those of which he is a part."[10] For an impressionable youngster, these
were important years.

While these would indeed prove the halcyon days of Lloyd's youth,
the bright future darkened shortly after the family's arrival. A nationwide financial panic brought the collapse of the Louisville-Covington
railway venture. This forced a move to humbler yet still comfortable
dwellings, a one-story frame structure. Despite this setback, both parents were well equipped to take care of themselves and their family.
Nelson returned to teaching and took engineering jobs during the summer months, including various surveying jobs building highways and
railways in northern Kentucky and the South. Sophia would add to the

family income as well by teaching, for despite the rural setting one local of the period admitted that in general "there was a feeling favorable to rudimentary education."[11]

While there is every indication that the Lloyds were relatively prosperous, like all families they experienced periods of hardship and times of joy.

These early days in northern Kentucky witnessed a Lloyd household on the move in search of opportunities. After Burlington, the family moved to Petersburg, then to Florence (both in Boone County), and later to Crittenden in Grant County, Kentucky. While in Florence the Lloyds added two more sons: Curtis Gates on July 17, 1859, and Robert Llewellyn on May 25, 1864. In addition Nelson and Sophia adopted a little girl named Emma, who became as close a member of the Lloyd family as any of the brothers.[12] On June 19, 1867, tragedy befell the family when "little Lewie" (Robert Llewellyn) died. The exact nature of his illness is unclear, but it has been alleged that John's baby brother was treated with a mustard plaster adulterated with flour by a druggist more interested in his profit than his product.[13] The efficacy of the prescribed "cure" is doubtful in any case. In an age when the etiology of disease was poorly understood, diagnosis and therapeutics were very often little more than guesswork; death's visitation to the Lloyd household typified an all too common event in nineteenth-century America. John probably took the sad event stoically, ascribing the passing of one so young to God's will; it was, after all, a time when nearly every youth expected the loss of a brother, sister, or parent.[14] Despite the loss, the family carried on.

The Florence years must have been some of John Uri Lloyd's happiest, for he memorialized them years later in his so-called Stringtown novels (see chapter 8). It was during this period that the fond memories of colorful characters spinning yarns captured a young boy's imagination. Yet it was his interest in the local flora and fauna that would set his future course. His fascination with nature turned to experimentation with a little gentle prodding from his parents. Fifty years later, the chairman of the education section of the American Pharmaceutical Association (APhA) asked Lloyd to write down his recollection of this early period in his life:

My apprenticeship in pharmacy may thus be said to have begun in my home years, for even when I was too young to be properly enrolled in the class in chemistry in the school, my interest in that subject was such that, when the class was reciting, I had thought for nothing else, and at home I was guided into home experiments, in which such exhibition substances as oxygen, hydrogen, etc., were made conspicuously entertaining. I of course had no apparatus, such as glass tubes or retorts, but the very lack of such appliances led me to exercise ingenuity in finding something to take their place. I well remember how connected stems of the pumpkin vine were made to furnish a delivery tube for gases generated in an old-fashioned, conical ink bottle, to a pneumatic trough improvised from my mother's quart camphor bottle being borrowed (surreptitiously), to collect the gases generated in my back-yard laboratory.[15]

When John reached the age of fourteen, his parents decided it was time to find their eldest son a position as a druggist's apprentice. The precise evolution of this educational plan is unclear, but it was undoubtedly facilitated by the lad's propensity to spirit away his mother's household appliances in the cause of "science." Undoubtedly the boy had shown a tendency toward inquiry and experimentation in his natural surroundings, something that two teacher-parents quickly noticed, encouraged, and indeed turned to their son's advantage. "They were united in the opinion that *thoroughness in preliminary work*, directly designed to fit one for a life vocation, was the first essential for success," Lloyd remembered, "and although they did not underrate the value of a college education and were in a financial position to send me to college, they feared that if my school education were made the first requisite, I would not be willing to begin at the bottom in pharmacy, a thing they believed to be essential in the training of a pharmacist, and that I would thus be diverted from my life work."[16]

John Uri Lloyd's explanation here is troublesome. Drawn from a 1915 perspective, it begs the question: Why become a pharmacist at all? Why, for example, did the Lloyds not direct their son toward a physician's life? The reason may have had to do with the status of the medical profession at the time. Cincinnati's *Medical Observer* noted in 1857, for example, that "It has become fashionable to speak of the Medical Profession as a body of jealous, quarrelsome men, whose chief delight is the annoyance and ridicule of each other."[17] Indeed for the country as a whole, doctors enjoyed none of the high rank accorded them in the twentieth century. "The prestige of the medical profession was scarcely high at the end of the eighteenth century," writes medical historian John Duffy, "and if any change occurred during the next fifty or sixty years, it was probably for the worse."[18] Although it is surprising from today's perspective, most physicians prior to World War I were men of modest means who had to supplement their incomes by farming or selling drugs.[19] Given this state of affairs, it is easy to see why observant parents would question the wisdom of such a field for their son. While pharmacy was barely a profession in the 1860s and hardly of high status, it was probably regarded by the general public as a comparatively honorable trade (as trades went at the time) affording most proprietors a reasonable return on their investment.

Other careers are more difficult to dismiss, however. Cincinnati (just a few miles north of the Lloyd family residence) offered ample opportunities for formal education in other fields.[20] Lawyers, for example, held prestigious positions in nineteenth-century America, and success in the legal profession very often provided the doorway to the powerful seats of government. Law had been taught at Cincinnati College since 1836, and few schools of higher education worthy of the name could not list law among their course offerings. A very real advantage to pursuing this line of education was the fact that the family already had connections with the legal profession in Sophia's brother, Edward Webster, an attorney in Rochester, New York. John Lloyd would not have been the first person to have his professional career materially aided by some kindly nepotism. Even excluding law, there remained any number of opportunities for instruction in the "mechanical arts" such as his father's own civil engineering, or design, architecture, and a variety of applied sciences. Most noteworthy of these was the Ohio Mechanic's Institute, first chartered in 1829 "for advancing the best interests of the mechanics, manufacturers, and artisans, by the more general diffusion of useful knowledge in those important classes of the community."[21] What better place for a civil engineer's son to receive instruction?

As Nelson Lloyd traveled throughout Kentucky, the engineer-teacher could not have helped but notice the many educational offerings available to his son in his own state. One of the more interesting and innovative was the Agricultural and Mechanical College, founded on February 22, 1865, as part of Kentucky University in Lexington. The president of the university at the time, John B. Bowman, was a great believer in a pragmatic education and insisted that all students work either on the college's experimental farm or in its "mechanical works" established in 1868, where such practical hands-on skills as carpentry and blacksmithing were taught as adjuncts to more traditional courses.[22]

The point is that with ample educational opportunities available both to the north and south, it is hard to imagine two well-educated and well-informed parents like Nelson and Sophia simply ignoring these possibilities. It is equally unlikely that as teachers themselves they were unaware of the sweeping alteration of American education and the implications that these changes would have for all their children. Abraham Lincoln's signing of the Morrill Act in 1862 caused "land grant" colleges like the A & M college in Lexington to dot the landscape almost immediately. Indeed, by the 1860s there were many influential forces at work centralizing and mandating formal education nationwide, not the least of which was the establishment of the United States Office of Education in 1867.[23]

John Uri Lloyd's explanation of his early education to members of the American Pharmaceutical Association in 1915, therefore, does not address the real question of why other avenues were not pursued by his parents. True, Lloyd had begun his apprenticeship before Kentucky's A & M college was founded, but with such vast practical educational innovations developing around him, why not abandon a future in the druggist's trade for this and perhaps other opportunities? Lloyd was, after all, only sixteen in 1865. It was a question that vexed Lloyd himself, and he was continually bringing the matter up throughout his life as if to rationalize his lack of formal instruction. In his autobiographical typescript (an unfinished, fragmentary manuscript produced late in his life and probably intended for eventual publication), Lloyd stated that he would not spend a great deal of time on the topic of his formal training "partly to *absolve my parents from neglect* [emphasis added] and partly to acquaint the reader with conditions at that time."[24] Lloyd goes on to state that "collegiate educations were markedly devoted to accomplishment in the line of finishing one for a more polished future, rather than to instruction along the lines of practical utility. They may be classed in the avocational sphere of life rather than the vocational." Lloyd is only half correct. True, the classical education that emphasized the ancient languages (Latin and/or Greek) along with philosophy and the other humanities (often including other refinements such as oratory and elocution) was the foundation of most college curricula of the period, but the many examples given in and around Lloyd's boyhood home of northern Kentucky show that even in the 1860s course offerings were expanding and practical studies were becoming more prevalent.

So why did John Lloyd not go to Lexington's A & M college, the Ohio Mechanic's Institute, or law school, or some other facility devoted to more career-oriented students? It is hard to say; any definitive evidence in his parents' correspondence is lacking or lost. But there are hints that perhaps young Johnny had little interest in or facility for more bookish pursuits. His uncle Edward Webster, no doubt with an attorney's eye for assessing character, apparently noticed this in Lloyd as a young man and commented on his nephew's lack of breadth. Dispensing some well-intentioned avuncular advice, he wrote to young John in 1869, "do not loose [sic] sight of the higher and more important interests of a future life. Do not either ignore literary studies & pursuits and if you can do so write for the papers occasionally for your own *intellectual* if not pecuniary profit."[25] What was in evidence at age twenty was probably demonstrated in John's earlier habits. While his homemade experiments show an inquisitive and inventive mind, there is no collateral evidence of sustained reading or a voracious appetite for more theoretical knowledge. All of the schools that offered practical training of some kind during this time would have also had core requirements more typical of traditional academia. Languages, history, philosophy, literature, and oratory all would have had some part in any reputable school's curriculum as an essential requisite for the "well-rounded" citizen. Lloyd's parents, undoubtedly adept at assessing the skills and potentials of children, must have pondered the likelihood of academic success in their son and opted for a future that offered financial security and social respectability without passing the hurdles of formal scholarship. Nelson and Sophia surely studied and searched for the proper career that would call upon John's natural curiosity and scientific propensities and yet avoid the propaedeutic requirements of traditional academics. Such an opportunity afforded itself in pharmacy.

Formal education in pharmacy in the United States was largely a post–Civil War development.[26] Early starts made in Philadelphia (1821), Massachusetts (1823), New York (1829), New Orleans (1838), Maryland (1840), and Chicago (1859) constituted the extent of available schooling in the field up until the war. Even these noble efforts, however, were often met with a lackluster response by most Americans. The Massachusetts College of Pharmacy, for example, gave lectures in the subject but was unable to launch regular course work until 1867. The result was there were fewer than five hundred pharmacists with diplomas prior to the Civil War.[27] Cincinnati's efforts began even later, with thirty-two matriculants in the 1871–1872 season and its first ten graduates in 1872–1873.[28] Indeed the 1870s, according to Glenn Sonnedecker, "marked a kind of turning point in education as it did in other areas of pharmaceutical activity." Nevertheless, in spite of the growth of pharmacy schools across the nation during the last third of the nineteenth century, a mere 12 percent of the practicing pharmacists in America had anything beyond an apprenticeship training in their field by century's end.[29]

Thus, as the young boy and his father set out for Cincinnati in the early morning hours during the late summer of 1863, the pursuit of an apprenticeship in pharmacy represented a career decision based upon the realistic assessment of young John's demonstrated abilities rather than the wishful thinking that no amount or number of tuition payments could fulfill. Central to that choice was a vocation that would call upon skills in the applied sciences rather than a diverse knowledge of the humanities or the study of broad theoretical principles. To their credit, Nelson Marvin and Sophia Webster Lloyd made a decision most likely to produce success rather than failure and frustration for their eldest son. Because John Uri Lloyd did not show any sustained interest or ability in academic work should not imply that he was an inept dunderhead; he simply was not of a scholarly bent. Nonetheless, his marked facility in practical and applied science would remain his strong suit throughout his life, and his naturally inquisitive nature would materially benefit the field of pharmacy in significant ways. First, however, a position had to be found. Lloyd's reminiscences of that time with his father in search of an apprenticeship were fondly recounted years later. It bears quoting at length because it shows not only the circumstances of his entry into the field of pharmacy but also the relationship that he had with his father, the picturesque life of a busy river city whose trade had returned to normal as the war neared its end, and the general state of the pharmaceutical business during the 1860s:

The boy seeking a position in far-off Cincinnati needed to start early, no time had he to linger until "stage time," nor would economy permit him such lavish extravagance as that fare demanded. To start at four o'clock in the morning in the milk wagon, or to walk to the city and back again was not a disagreeable task to either my father or myself. Indeed the foot journey during the pleasant summer time appealed, inasmuch as father's conversation was so instructively entertaining as to make the journey a pleasure, it could have been longer to the boy's advantage. Arriving in Covington [in Kentucky opposite Cincinnati] by the milk wagon about 5 o'clock in the morning would have been too early for business establishments to be open, but the time between was not lost. Mother would have prepared a breakfast about half past three which fortified us until noon and each trip father had something of interest to show me in the great city I hoped to make my future.

The first morning we walked to the Suspension Bridge over the Licking River [not to be confused with the John A. Roebling bridge across the Ohio completed in 1866], between Covington and Newport. He explained its construction, gave me the history of suspension bridges in general, embellishing the story with an account of Blondin's feat of wire walking across [the] Niagara River in 1859. This he did most vividly, finally saying, "Johnny, this Newport–Covington Suspension Bridge should be of particular interest to you because your father located the piers on which the structure rests. When I came to survey a railway line between Covington and Louisville, the contractors needed the exact location of these piers. I took my company of engineers and made the survey for them." This incident is related to indicate that time was not long to the boy seeking a business location, indeed the time when the drug stores began to open their doors seemed to come very soon. Then we began on the errand of the day. From one apothecary shop to another we trudged, the question at each being—"Do you need a boy?" I doubt if we missed a Covington establishment, but no vacancy was found. . . .

These trips were taken each Saturday in the early autumn and early winter of 1864, and as I look back [I] can comprehend they were not designed alone to obtain a drug store position. Affairs of life were discussed as opportunity presented, indeed in certain instances attempts to find a situation were secondary. For example, nearly a day was lost in a visit to the Cincinnati Water Works and reservoir on the hillside above where great machinery proved a wonder to the boy from Kentucky. . . .

Again he would take me to the river front where on the levee was a scene of marvelous activity. Cotton bales by the thousand, sugar, molasses, resin by the acre, were being unloaded from the steamers from the South.[30] Elsewhere like amounts of flour, bacon, barreled pork, whisky, machinery and manufactured goods of every description were being stored awaiting their turn to be drayed to the steamers unloading supplies from the South. Only space sufficient for the movements of the horse vehicles and winding avenues for foot persons was available. . . .

We had vainly searched the city of Covington, had crossed the river to Cincinnati and had begun again the new old story—"Do you need a boy?" From one drug store to another we passed, sometimes pleasantly received, sometimes snappishly. Once or twice the apothecary patted me on the head in a sympathetic manner but more often I received but a passing glance as came the familiar word, "No."

Systematically did we take the city, beginning at the river and progressing backward. Every store between Millcreek on the left and Deercreek on the right was visited as we wedged back towards the hills. In one instance an apothecary in a small store on the western edge of the city encouraged us with the hope that next Saturday he might have a vacancy as the present boy was "thinking of quitting." But by the next Saturday the boy had decided to remain. This was a mighty disappointment because the apothecary had discussed at some length the problem of pharmacy and its opportunities, but not giving a very encouraging aspect to the business as a life vocation. Said he: "Long hours, few vacations, the work slavish, all business. Better find something else for the boy." "Good advice," said my father, as we started for the next store, "but it does not always seem to apply. To stop now would be to give up because of discouragements. Not until we find there is no chance will we turn to some other business."

At last at the corner of Eighth Street and Western Row (now Central Avenue) [at] a very extensive establishment, the proprietor (my father always asked for the proprietor) said that he expected soon to need a boy as one of his boys expected to leave soon. He exhibited much interest in our affairs, asked a multitude of questions, quizzed me personally concerning myself, then summed it up to the effect that we might possibly well continue our search for a situation as it might be some weeks before his position opened. The firm name was W. J. M. Gordon & Brother. The next drug store visited was two squares away, at the corner of Court and Plum Streets. Here the proprietor, whom I afterward found was Mr. H. M. Merrell, answered "Yes." He needed a boy. Elated at the final success, a tentative agreement was made with the understanding that I was to begin the next week. The firm name was H. M. Merrell & Co. Back to Gordon we went elated over our success. To our surprise Mr. Gordon said that will never do if you expect to become a druggist in Cincinnati. The house is not in good standing among us. It is an "Eclectic" establishment without professional affiliations. To take that situation will be to destroy your future. Much more did Mr. Gordon say, enough to lead my father to decide that for my sake it would be best to decline the position we had so long sought. Back to Mr. Merrell we went and at once my father presented the case exactly as he knew it. Said he, "The boy needs to become a prescription clerk in a general drug store. I am informed that your establishment is intimately connected with a section in medicine and pharmacy that would not give the boy general prescription opportunities." To this Mr. Merrell agreed, stating that he had no prescription business to speak of, that he needed a boy to run errands and do chores, but not to learn the prescription business. And he advised us to wait until we could get the position offered by Mr. Gordon where no better educational opportunities in pharmacy could be had in all Cincinnati.

Mr. Gordon seemed pleased with our decision and unexpectedly stated that he would give me a position at once as he could use both boys to advantage. It was therefore decided that the next Saturday I would begin my work. This was in the late fall of 1863.[31]

A position had been found. Now would come the process of making John Uri Lloyd a pharmacist. But it was more than that: it was also the beginning of the evolution of a wide-eyed boy from rural Boone County, Kentucky, into a man of science and business. Lloyd's apprenticeship was a major metamorphosis, the transformation from a rustic dilettante who concocted improvised experiments at home to a compounding pharmacist who would eventually become an innovative researcher who helped move the preparation of medicines from an inexact, willy-nilly affair to one of higher standards of purity, strength, and greater uniformity and reliability.

One cannot leave this early period in the life of John Lloyd without the distinct impression that he in many ways personified larger changes at work in America at the time. Just as Lloyd himself was on the brink of casting off the rough eccentricities of his bucolic provincialism in exchange for the wider vision necessary for a man with much larger projects, so too was the nation at large. The triumph of union over secession in 1865 set the nation on a new course, with a new spirit animating virtually every aspect of society. Lloyd's family was remarkably unaffected by the war. None of the Lloyd brothers went to war, and relatives do not appear to have openly engaged in the conflict. Although surprisingly little mention is made of the war in family correspondence, Lloyd's father was angered at being forced to give an oath of allegiance to the Union and quietly sympathized with the South. Every American of this generation had *some* opinion of the conflict, and Lloyd's attitudes would be revealed years later in his Stringtown novels (see chapter 8). Overall, however, the Lloyd family (like many in northern Kentucky) chiefly wished to remain neutral and for the fighting to stop.

Nevertheless, John Uri Lloyd was caught up in the larger forces of urbanization and industrialization ushered in by the war. As young John took his apprenticeship under Gordon, he was launched upon a vast wave of social, political, economic, and scientific change, the crest of which he would ride to great heights of accomplishment and acclaim. First, however, he would have to bear life's inevitable rites of passage, an initiation process that would take place in the dynamic atmosphere of the Queen City.

2

The Rustic Apprentice,
1864–1870

✍ The city that John Uri Lloyd entered in late 1863 was a bustling metropolis of 186,329 men, women, and children. Like Rome, this "Queen of the West" had grown surrounded by seven hills. Thus, early Cincinnati was confined to a small section of the Ohio River Basin. As these girdling hills became settled in the latter third of the nineteenth century, they received the names by which they are known today: to the east lay Mt. Adams, Mt. Lookout, and Mt. Washington; to the west, Price's Hill and Mt. Airy; to the north, Mt. Auburn and Mt. Healthy. When young John arrived, the establishment of these stylish suburbs peopled by the city's emerging middle and upper classes was just around the corner. For now (the early 1860s) Cincinnati remained a "walking city" (or perhaps more accurately, a running, pushing, and jostling city), where virtually all citizens lived within a pedestrian's distance of home, work, school, church, or synagogue. The natural topography of the area accentuated the activity and congestion of the city by cramming well over thirty thousand people per square mile into the mere 3.88 available in the valley, making it one of the most densely packed urban centers of the United States.[1]

Friedrich Ratzel, a German scientist-tourist during the period of Lloyd's early apprenticeship who had visited St. Louis, Chicago, and Cincinnati, left a vivid and rather detailed account of the "most venerable among these young queens."[2] It was a city constrained by hills and bounded by a river whose ever-growing factories belched out smoke and fumes that contributed to a "murky, soot-filled atmosphere." The noxious fumes coming from above were mixed with the odors of the ever-present fecal matter from below as the incessant pig drives through town to the meat-packing plants left their undeniable mark on "Porkopolis." At its worst, the stench and cacophony must have seemed like the very bowels of hell. Ratzel pointed out, however, that some semblance of order was provided by streets "evenly laid out as far as topography allows": those running east-west being numbered; those running north-south having mainly common botanical names such as Vine, Plum, Elm, and Sycamore. The unpleasantries were also ameliorated by many "handsome granite and sandstone buildings," which lent an air of elegance and prosperity to the surroundings.

As John and his father walked the city streets, they could not have helped but notice the conspicuous class stratifications and diversity in the expanding city. Comfortable and often elaborate homes were located in the heart of downtown. Fourth Street, Garfield Place, and Dayton Street in the so-called West End provided a plush respite from the flurry of commercial life for Cincinnati's elite. Least desirable were the slums of Deer Creek Valley east of the city and the riverfront area called Rat Row where street toughs looked for easy marks and prostitutes catered to the ever-present roustabouts. Between these two extremes were tens of thousands of hardworking and industrious Germans who had poured into the city during the 1830s and 1840s. By mid-century, German was nearly as commonly heard on the streets as was English. In some pockets of the city like Over-the-Rhine, one could scarcely distinguish the neighborhood from any in Germany itself.[3] In 1863 Cincinnati was a kaleidoscope of socioeconomic and ethnic variation: it was a hardworking, moneymaking, money-taking, high-living, river-faring, sausage-eating, beer-drinking, German-speaking city in perpetual motion.

To a boy of fourteen from Kentucky, the buzz of urban life must have offered an exciting—sometimes frightening—contrast to his former pastoral surroundings. The sight of a countrified youth in the big city would not have been unusual, however, as people (especially the young) began to leave the farms for the excitement and opportunities that urban centers offered. Yet America was a nation still three-quarters rural; of all the cities or towns in the United States at the time, only eleven had populations of more than fifty thousand.[4] As one of the few truly large metropolitan areas in the United States at the time, Cincinnati was drawing in many youths in search of fame and fortune. John Lloyd was surely not the only rustic apprentice in town.

The pharmacist under whom Lloyd would study was anything but typical.[5] His full name was William John Maclester Gordon, born in Somerset County, Maryland, on Christmas Day, 1825. He had apprenticed under his cousin in Baltimore, and in addition he took formal course work in chemistry at the University of Maryland before coming to Cincinnati in 1848. The firm, under the company name W.J.M. Gordon and Brother, was well known in the area, and its proprietor was respected as a reliable wholesale druggist, described as "ambitious, persevering, energetic and capable." Always active in the American Pharmaceutical Association, founded in 1852, he was elected its twelfth president in 1864.

The business that young John was apprenticed to in 1863 was quite active and lucrative. One of Gordon's chief sources of profit was the manufacture of glycerin, the first operation of its kind west of the Allegheny mountains.[6] Colorless and odorless with a warm, sweetish taste, glycerin's benefits were touted by Gordon as a soothing and healing topical for chapped skin and hands, as a stable vehicle in "remedies for both internal and external use," as a preservative in cerates and ointments, and dozens of other uses. Gordon was well situated to produce glycerin since his proximity to the great soap and candle company, Procter and Gamble, gave him a ready supply of the "sweet water" necessary to glycerin production. Procter and Gamble, happy to rid itself of this unwanted fatty byproduct produced by hydrolysis of its soap-making process, freely gave Gordon all the sweet water he needed. All that Gordon really needed to do was purify the material through distillation with steam. The final glycerin that Gordon sold for $1.25 per pound, therefore, represented virtually total profit.

But Lloyd was apprenticed to Gordon to learn much more than the glycerin business; he was to learn pharmacy from the bottom up. Thus, specific arrangements had to be arrived at that were clear and mutually understood at the outset. Toward that end, it was agreed that Lloyd would be under Gordon's charge for two years; he was to be paid $2 per week for the first six months, with fifty-cent increases for the next two six-month periods; and he would receive $4 per week for the last six months.[7] Comparisons are always risky and tenuous at best, but if J. F. Hancock's experience in Baltimore in 1854 is any indication (he appears to have been a typical druggist's apprentice of the period), the terms under which Lloyd worked were quite reasonable. Hancock struck a verbal agreement with Dr. J. L. Large to study under him at a salary of $25 for the first six months with incremental increases up to a total of $800 for an entire four-year term.[8] In comparison, Lloyd (at his agreed-upon two-year rate, with fifty-cent increases up to four years) would have grossed a total of $780 for the same period. The similarity in these two figures from two different urban centers is striking in a field that at the time lacked statutory regulation or standardization.

In reference to his apprenticeship under Gordon, Lloyd speaks of his humiliatingly "small pay," but his complaint must be set in the context of the times. While $2 a week was indeed a low wage even by 1860s standards, it must be recognized that for Lloyd, who also received his board, it was not much under the pay scales of some other workers who received board. Mill workers in a New Haven factory, for example, earned an average of $2.60 per week, as did the typical hired farmhand who worked eight months out of the year for an average of $2.34 per week.[9] Indeed Lloyd the apprentice would outstrip both the mill worker and farm laborer by his second year. Lloyd's wages were not all that bad considering that he was just a student preparing himself to make considerably greater income with a future in pharmacy. In so doing, he would first have to learn the requisite skills of the apothecary art as it existed in the 1860s.

What exactly was the present state of pharmacy in the United States at that time? The answer to this question is important because it establishes the nature and extent of Lloyd's early training and the prospects for his future. The first thing to be said about pharmaceutical practice in America at this time is that, like most areas of commercial and public life, it was overwhelmingly dominated by men. Up to the Civil War, female practitioners in pharmacy were practically unheard of. Although wartime shortages of manpower forced some druggists to hire women as clerk assistants, the prevailing cult of domesticity kept most women out of the field on a more permanent basis. By 1870, observes Teresa Catherine Gallagher, "34 women and 17,335 men were recorded as traders and dealers in drugs and medicines."[10]

Of more immediate significance to Lloyd was pharmacy's transitional status in the 1860s. Prior to the Civil War, pharmacies had largely been businesses operated by physicians and sometimes sold to their clerks. This encouraged a situation in which the apothecary's skills and practices were considered a simple trade to be pursued as profits dictated. Because of this unprofessional attitude, pharmacy was frequently part of a general sundries supply that not uncommonly evolved into an unintentional wholesale operation.[11] By the Civil War, however, pharmaceutical practice was undergoing tremendous change. The establishment of the American Pharmaceutical Association in 1852 did much to set the discipline on a truly professional course. Also, the open, laissez-faire environment in which virtually every component of the pharmacist's practice from drug purity standards to dispensing activities was left only to professional ethics was nearing its end. Although nationwide regulation would wait until the next century, the founding of state pharmacy associations sparked a flurry of state regulatory legislation during the last third of the nineteenth century.[12] All of these factors plus the impending impact of industrialization upon commercial pharmacy placed John Uri Lloyd in a truly watershed period.

The state of pharmaceutical education has already been noted in chapter 1, but what literature would Lloyd have studied during his apprenticeship? By today's standards the American source materials available to Lloyd as an apprentice in pharmacy were quite meager.[13] First there was the *Practical Pharmacy: The Arrangements, Apparatus and Manipulations of the Pharmaceutical Shop*, published in 1849 by William Procter Jr. (1817–1874), a professor of pharmacy at the Philadelphia College of Pharmacy. In addition, there was Edward Parrish's *Introduction to Practical Pharmacy* (1856). To augment these texts, there were the published annual *Proceedings of the American Pharmaceutical Association* and the *American Journal of Pharmacy*, which had been formed largely through the efforts of Procter, the period's most eminent figure in American pharmacy.[14] For ongoing practical advice and collegial information, there was always the *Druggist's Circular*, first issued in 1857.

As important as any of these items might have been during the period, nothing symbolized the growing professionalization of the field more than the *Pharmacopeia of the United States of America (USP)* and the *United States Dispensatory (USD)*. First published in 1820, the *USP* represented the combined efforts of Samuel Latham Mitchell (1764–1831) and Lyman Spalding (1775–1821) to produce a compendium of preparations and drugs of generally agreed upon (though sometimes arguable) efficacy. The reference sources were designed to standardize practice and serve as a guide to the appropriate materia medica and nomenclature to be applied by pharmacists.[15] In other words, the USP was supposed to serve as the druggist's guide to those manufactured "officinals" that should be kept on hand at all times as well as the proper "preparations and compositions" to be compounded by him. Lloyd's entry into pharmacy coincided with the fourth revision of the USP, and its great popularity necessitated a second printing by 63.[16] Despite this fact, it was the *Dispensatory*, authored by two eminent physicians, Franklin Bache (1792–1864) and George B. Wood (1797–1879), both of the Philadelphia College of Pharmacy, which in historian Gregory Higby's words, "became the most popular American medical reference book of the century."[17] More than just a compendium of names and preparations, the USD contained commentary and explanations of material found in the USP. Thus, from the perspective of the student and druggist, the USD became the bible of every American apothecary. The practical value of the USD in Lloyd's early days in pharmacy can hardly be overstated. "Rather than view the USD as some popularization or replacement for the pharmacopoeia," writes Higby, "we should recognize it for what it effectively was—the de facto guide of pharmacy practice during the middle half of the 1800s. To thousands of pharmacists and physicians, the dispensatory *was* the pharmacopoeia."[18] These, then, were the printed tools available during John Uri Lloyd's apprenticeship.

Lloyd's own description of his training under Gordon reveals an approach to the discipline that undoubtedly involved some of the materials discussed above but primarily focused on the student's ability to memorize and learn by example:

> In the line of real pharmacy came, after some months, the reading of prescriptions, and the learning of the tables of weights and measures, with their uses. Standing by the side of the head clerk when he filled prescriptions, I watched him make the compounds, and had the reasons for the various mix-

tures explained to me. At last I was permitted to make the measurements for simple prescriptions, such as a mixture of Syrup of Squills with Syrup of Ipecac, and pour the mixture into the bottle, whilst Mr. Riefsnider watched the process, wrote the label, and numbered the prescription. I was drilled in the rolling of pills and in the selection of excipients [i.e., binding agents such as honey or gum arabic used in pills], in the making of the medicinal syrups then in use, and in the beginning of pharmacy, as pharmacy was then practiced. That was the day of heroic medication [i.e., a therapeutic system involving the blistering, bleeding, and purging of patients]. The spreading of plasters was continuous, and that process I soon learned. I would give much now [Lloyd was writing in 1915 here] for the old "Plaster Iron" I so frequently used in making the "Strengthening Plasters," "Diachylon Plaster," and above all, "Blistering Plasters," (Canthrides), to fit different parts of the body, such as the back of the neck, or behind the ears, all these being with us, constant necessities. In these rudiments, by reason of the help and advice continually given me by my preceptors, I soon became proficient, and when my two years of apprenticeship had passed, I found myself capable, in the absence of other clerks, of waiting upon the front store, and of "selling" simples, such as "senna and manna," epsom salts, and other remedies called for over the counter, and even of compounding simple prescriptions, where there was no question as to my understanding of the same. By this time I had learned to make emulsions, to compound pills by means of the best excipients, to make suppositories with paper cones, in the old-fashioned way. In fact, I was fairly proficient, for an apprentice of two years' experience. I was also taught that I must become conversant with the natures of drugs, and especially of the poisons. I was taught, verbally, the qualities of the different agents, and I put all my spare time, (none too abundant), in reading the Dispensatory. My chief opportunity for study came on Sunday, for on that day no business was permitted in Mr. Gordon's establishment, other than the compounding of prescriptions and the dispensing of legitimate medicines. No toilet articles were sold; no soaps, no soda drinks, nothing outside of medicine formed a part of our Sunday business.[19]

Lloyd's own experience shows the importance of practical hands-on experience and the preeminence of the *USD* in the druggist's life of the mid-nineteenth century.

But an apprentice had much more to learn than the drug business; he had to learn some of life's lessons. These would be taught eagerly (if less systematically) by his own peers. Although Lloyd was the only apprentice in the Gordon drugstore, the proprietor had several other boys under his employ as regular workers. Johnny became a ready source of amusement for these lads because of his small size (always smaller than that of other boys his own age), his attachment to his homespun shawl, and his country ways. Lloyd's behavior (undoubtedly viewed as eccentric) got him singled him out for special attention, and the young Kentuckian became the butt of several harmless but humiliating jokes. They would soak his drinking straw in quinine, giving his favorite lemon soda a bitter taste. Since he was familiar only with the general stores of northern Kentucky, which carried virtually everything, the boys took advantage of Lloyd's naiveté and sent him to specialty houses for items they did not carry; or sometimes they simply taunted him. John took it all in stride, and he admitted years later that these rites of passage, though hard at the time, forced him to rely upon his own resources and "I was made to take care of myself."[20]

When young John was not facing these peer pressures he, like all apprentices of the period, had to deal with the sheer drudgery of life in a drugstore. Lloyd's day began at seven in the morning, with the first order of business being his trip to the post office to take and receive the store's mail. Besides this, he was expected "to sweep the store, clean up the soda counter, wash all the glasses, wash the bottles for the prescription counter and case, clean the graduates and mortars used in compounding prescriptions, once a week wash all the windows, run errands as necessity required, fill the soda syrups and wait on the soda counter, and at odd times, put in my time filling and folding Seidlitz Powders [i.e., a mild laxative composed of tartaric acid and a mixture of sodium bicarbonate and Rochelle salt]."[21]

Lloyd's portrayal of his apprenticeship under Gordon is cast as if it were especially beneficial in part because of its severity. Yet others experienced much the same. J. F. Hancock was assigned very similar duties in Baltimore, and William Dupont's apprenticeship "program" at the H. and L. Simoneau store in Detroit included "all manner of chores." Dupont recalled that "The grinding, powdering of drugs, roots, herbs, gums, etc., was part of his duties."[22] For that matter, life in the mid-nineteenth-century drugstore was hard and unglamorous *at all levels*. Writing in 1907, A. E. Magoffin remembered these harsh realities as he recounted his experiences during the "good old days" of the drug business in Bainbridge, Ohio:

One of my first duties in the drug life was the making of tinctures, syrups, etc. I can shut my eyes now and look back to the later fifties [Magoffin would have been about thirteen or fourteen years old] and see a row of half-gallon and one-gallon specie jars sitting on a shelf in our back room, and am reminded of the seven and fourteen day maceration periods—then straining through a cloth (no filter paper then that I call to mind). How I'd squeeze and squeeze those cloths to get out all the liquid. We knew nothing of tincture presses.

A wonderful difference has made itself evident in these fifty years. We saved not only six to thirteen days in manufacture, but also a large amount of loss by evaporation, as well as a lot of hard and tedious work.

Then I can recall the luscious compound cathartic pill—that good old-fashioned cure-all for everything but amputated legs. My stunt was usually 2,000 every month, sometimes oftener. My! Oh, my! How I hated that job; and while I am writing I may say I am tasting the colocynth—whew! how nasty. No sugar-coating in ours, then, thank you; just plain pill, taste included. Along in 1871 or 1872 I bought a small sugar-coater, guaranteed to coat 200 pills at a time, but it was no good.

Then I remember that old—not sachet—powder called "hicry picry" by our patrons [probably a play on words for Hiera Picra (powders of aloes and canella), a popular unofficial preparation with an extremely bitter flavor]. How's that for taste in the mouth, you old fellows? Do you recall it? I do almost as good as "fetty" [probably asafetida, an herb yielding a gummy resin with an exceptionally bad odor and taste]. I ground my own spices up till about 1874. In fact, I did so in the eighties, and guaranteed them pure.[23]

Lloyd pursued his training with admirable tenacity. Realizing that two years' apprenticeship was not enough to become proficient at pharmacy, he next went to George Eger (1836–1900) "an accomplished German pharmacist" located along Cincinnati's canal on the west side. For a two-year term at $3 per week plus board, Lloyd advanced his studies.

Eger, like Gordon, had above-average credentials as an apprentice's instructor. His training and early career were spent in Esslingen and Stuttgart, Germany, and Geneva, Switzerland. After coming to America in 1855, he practiced in Terre Haute, Indiana, and St. Louis, Missouri, before returning to Europe to study at the University of Tübingen. Eger was elected president of the Cincinnati College of Pharmacy several times, and he served as one of its trustees and on lecture and examination committees of the college.

While life at Eger's establishment included much the same mindless toil that Lloyd had experienced under Gordon such as sweeping floors, washing windows, and cleaning apparatus, it did include some important additions. Under Eger's charge, for example, Lloyd had the opportunity of attending chemistry lectures delivered by the eminent physician Roberts Bartholow (1831–1904) at the Medical College of Ohio. Eger's instruction also appears to have continued much of Gordon's teaching but in a somewhat more intensive and systematized manner. "As an apprentice with Mr. Eger," writes Lloyd, "I studied each night, beginning at eight o'clock, the Dispensatory record of some drug selected by him. The next night I wrote from memory a description of that drug, including its origin and history, its uses and doses, and if a poison, its antidote. The next evening he would review what I had written the previous night, criticizing and correcting it, emphasizing oversights. Then another drug was named, to be studied in like manner."[24]

At the conclusion of this two-year stint with Eger, the teacher pronounced John Uri Lloyd "competent to engage anywhere as a prescription clerk" with a written recommendation that would serve the graduate apprentice as his credentials to practice the apothecary arts. Interestingly, Lloyd returned to Gordon's store at Eighth and Central Avenues. At first he served as a "supernumerary clerk" without pay simply for the experience, but within a few weeks a position opened as assistant clerk and Lloyd was hired at $6 a week, soon raised to $10 per week. For an entry level position, this was reasonable (though by no means large) compensation. Although still below an average lower-middle-class family's annual income of $750 to $2,000, Lloyd's initial pay exceeded the average teacher's salary of the period by $10 per month.[25]

This time, however, it was not W. J. M. Gordon but rather Gordon's brother for whom Lloyd would work. During his apprenticeship with George Eger, the Gordons split the business, with William taking the lucrative glycerin factory in Deer Creek and his brother O. T. Gordon operating the drugstore on the northeast corner of Eighth Street and Central Avenue where Lloyd had first been introduced to the druggist's trade. It was during this period that Lloyd's younger brother Nelson Ashley (now nearly eighteen) was brought into the store on February 19, 1869. In order to help O. T. Gordon's flagging business, the brothers decided to initiate a "Department of Chemical Apparatus." They believed that the introduction of basic chemistry classes in the area's high schools would provide a ready market for such goods. Nevertheless, the Lloyds' well-intentioned efforts failed to revive the drugstore. O. T. Gordon could not maintain the business and was forced to assign the store operations over to his father-in-law and brother William to satisfy his creditors, but both men recognized the Lloyd brothers' interest in their chemical apparatus as a separate entity and allowed them a fair return on their inventory. While the store was still not on a sound financial footing and would eventually be forced to close permanently, at least for John and Ashley immediate disaster had been averted.

Lloyd speaks of the ending of his apprenticeship and his entry into the drug business as a clerk as if there were little or no break in his climb up the pharmaceutical ladder. In other words, Lloyd's published reminiscences suggest that he marched straight from George Eger's store to Gordon's, but there are clear indications of some sidetracks along the way. Lloyd's activities during this murky period between his release from Eger's apprenticeship in 1867 and his arrangement with Mr. Gordon is largely chronicled in his diaries.[26] Lloyd's very first diary entry dated September 21, 1867, indicates that he was with his father's surveying party in Kentucky near the Cumberland River. In fact all through the remainder of that year and on into 1868 his diary is riddled with entries leading with "in camp" or "moved camp." Whether John's father was merely putting his son to some meaningful work while he was between jobs or was seriously testing the youth's possible interest in engineering, it does appear that Nelson Marvin *did* get an impression as to the latter. In a letter to Sophia in the spring of 1868, he admitted, "I think John is getting enough of engineering and would be glad to get back into a drug store, but Ashley is enjoying it highly yet, he says he has gained six pounds since he left home."[27] John had had his fill of camp life. Shortly thereafter, indeed throughout the summer of that year, nineteen-year-old John was either doing odd jobs around his parent's house or simply "at home doing nothing." Finally on August 10, 1868, Lloyd wrote, "Went to Gordon's and begun work." This begins a long stretch of entries headed simply "On duty" or "At the store."

Besides Lloyd's work activities, these diary entries show the interests of a typical youth. While at home in Kentucky, Lloyd tended to chores, went to church, and visited with friends. As with most young men, women were catching his eye. One entry dated Sunday, May 8, 1870, includes a pressed flower with the words, "remember Nannie Poor," followed by a somewhat sketchy entry that recounts his daylong visit with the Poors and ends with "had a very pleasant time." Even when he was in Cincinnati, he maintained an active interest in his family back home and visited relatives in the city. There are frequent notations of his spending the day with "Uncle Dick and Aunt Eunice," his father's sister and her husband.

Although Lloyd took time to relax, work and business clearly predominate in his daily entries, and by the end of 1870 John's diary indicates that he and Ashley were ready to leave Gordon to start their own business. On December 8, 1870, appears the following entry: "Today Ashley and I rented a room on Broadway to commence manufacturing chemicals on the 1st of Jan., 1871. . . . Hope we will get along well and make a living. The lease runs one year and was signed and witnessed today." After giving notice to Gordon, both looked hopefully to a bright future. But less than three weeks after signing their lease, the unexpected happened. Lloyd wrote that, after escorting his aunt Eunice home, "this morning on my way back I tried to get upon the [street] cars while in motion, slipped and got my foot crushed under the wheels. Went back to Dick and had to have my big toe taken off. Women will be the death of me yet." The rest of the entries for that year read "Oh Oh Oh how it hurts," "At Dicks—Ache—Ache—All day, all night," "Oh what a foot—Aching all the time," and so on. The business venture collapsed. At best it would take John weeks to assume a normal routine; neither he nor his brother could afford to keep their manufacturing concern idle awaiting a recovery of uncertain duration. Nothing more is stated by John concerning the incident, and both brothers were apparently fortunate enough to get out of the lease without difficulty.

Despite these culs-de-sac in Lloyd's career, the 1870s would prove important years of advancement in his professional life. Although statutory regulations were few during that period, Lloyd passed the examination of Ohio's first qualifying body for pharmaceutical practitioners, the Cincinnati Pharmacy Board, organized in 1873. Of greater significance, however, was the fact that his position as a clerk at Gordon's store put him in an atmosphere conducive to making important contacts with the city's medical profession. Here Lloyd would experience the active interchange of personalities and exchange of ideas between the prescribing physicians and the drug clerks working at the store.

Chief among these contacts was his meeting with John King (1813–1894), a well-known eclectic physician. After witnessing the young man's attention to detail and single-minded devotion to his preparations, King offered Lloyd an unusual opportunity. "Dr. Scudder [King's eclectic colleague] and I have been discussing the necessity of the systematic study of our materia medica," Lloyd recalled of King's words to him, "as well as the re-study of our pharmaceutical preparations, both of which are now of vital importance. We have decided that you are the man to accept this responsibility, and for this purpose I am empowered to offer you the position of chemist with Mr. H. M. Merrell, with whom we have discussed the matter, and will, if you so agree, talk with you over the details. Before you decide," King ominously added, "you must consider the problem as a whole."[28] Such an offer clearly astonished Lloyd. An established and respected physician was asking the young man to make a decision destined to set the course of his professional life.

It must have been quite a sight. The bulky, 225-pound King (at fifty-seven, one of the icons of eclecticism) looking every bit the bearded sage, offering to the slender, five-foot, four-inch young man of twenty-one years an opportunity to enter the very heart of eclectic practice—its pharmacy. The embodiment of power and leadership stood beside youthful promise. Lloyd stood at a crossroads.

3

The Lure of Eclecticism

The problem that John King wanted Lloyd to consider "as a whole" was eclecticism and the costs that the young drug clerk would incur by associating with a sectarian or "irregular" school of medicine. In order to make sense of Lloyd's dilemma, it is necessary to understand the developmental context of eclecticism as a whole.

Even as late as the 1870s, there was no sharp line of demarcation between sectarian, or irregular medicine, and allopathy, or so-called regular medicine. This was in large part due to the fact that the fundamental tenets of modern medicine as it is understood today were only beginning to emerge in the nineteenth century. "The consequence of this was that science did matter to doctors collectively," writes historian W. F. Bynum, "even if it could be neglected by them individually, and even if much of ordinary medicine was untouched by it. There are three concrete aspects where this can be seen: medical education, professional identity, and the technology of medical practice."[1] It is, in fact, against these three benchmarks that most sectarian practice would fall behind, a liability that would eventually prove lethal. But these benchmarks depend upon the establishment of solid paradigms formed around clearly definable scientific principles; until these were firmly in place, measurable standards of comparison, except in the most extreme cases, are more difficult to gauge. For this reason, to speak of nineteenth-century medical practice in the United States as simply divided between regular physicians and unmitigated quacks is inaccurate presentism. As Abraham Flexner correctly noted in his classic study on medical education, "Prior to the placing of medicine on a scientific basis, sectarianism was, of course, inevitable. Every one started with some preconceived notion; and from a logical point of view, one preconception is as good as another."[2] Rival systems of medicine vied for supremacy, often engaging in vituperation and invective more than logic and objectivity. In such an environment, even the most eccentric and idiosyncratic notions had their say.

Within this milieu emerged the semiliterate figure of Samuel Thomson (1769–1843) with his *New Guide to Health; or Botanic Family Physician* in 1822.[3] Infused with large doses of the Galenic theory of restoring humoral balance within the body, Thomson's book argued for herbal remedies (especially lobelia) and an end to the bleeding and massive doses of calomel (mercurous chloride) common to "fashionable" doctors.[4] With Thomson's book of numbered botanical remedies, people were supposed to be able to diagnose and treat themselves after purchasing his patented system from an authorized agent for twenty dollars. Thomson's appeal to the masses was powerful because it bestowed upon everyone the alleged ability to heal themselves apart from the pretensions of the allopathic physician. Such a therapeutic system resonated with a Jacksonian democracy attempting to divest itself of what it viewed as elitist European notions that skill and knowledge are reserved only for those of rank and privilege.

At the same time, however, Thomson's system had fatal flaws. Thinking that the practice of medicine could substitute common sense for formal education, Samuel Thomson denied himself the institutional cohesiveness, collective strength, and financial advantages that a network of proprietary Thomsonian schools would have afforded. With everyone "practicing medicine" for twenty dollars and a book, personal attachments to the movement were weak and transient. Agents, likewise, tended to perform more as self-interested salesmen than disinterested disciples of the Thomsonian healing arts. Eventually, it became clear that Thomson had lost control over his system. "I am glad to hear that you scrupously *[sic]* adhere to the principles I have laid down in my *New Guide* for the treatment of disease. I have been informed," Thomson complained in 1837 to R. K. Frost "that this is not the case with many of the practitioners in the State of New York. They are taking my system out of the hands of the people, and are doing it an essential injury."[5] The problem was more widespread than just New York. Ultimately, Thomson's botanical movement was replaced by those better organized and more eager to create schools advocating his principles; they developed into a group identified by historian Alex Berman as the neo-Thomsonians.[6]

Another American medical sect was eclecticism. Unlike homeopathy, founded by the German physician Samuel Hahnemann (1755–1843), or hydropathy, founded by the Silesian peasant Vincenz Priessnitz (1790–1851), eclecticism had uniquely American roots.[7] It grew out of a larger grassroots movement spawned by the egalitarianism of Jacksonian democracy in the late 1820s through the 1830s. With a populace convinced of the innate wisdom of the masses, the superiority of all things American, and the complete bankruptcy of Old World ideas and institutions, a jingoistic fervor swept across the new nation with the intensity of a religious revival. These sociopolitical ideas translated into a nativist medical practice that sought to divest itself of the bleeding, blistering, and purging heroics of the allopaths.[8]

The eclectics were by far the most respectable and long-lived among the botanical groups, and they were medicine's self-styled popular protestant reformers.[9] This movement was started by Wooster Beach (1794–1868) under the rubric of "reformed medicine." As its name would imply, eclecticism held to no particular set of medical beliefs. "We have chosen, we are choosing, and we shall continue to choose those means which experience and experiment have proven and will prove curative,"[10] declared John Milton Scudder in 1889. This diffuse approach to medicine opened the eclectic movement to severe criticism. Comparing them with other sectarian groups, the *Medical and Surgical Reporter* noted in 1859 that "All the 'ics,' 'tics,' 'lics,' 'isms,' 'cisms,' 'ists,' and 'pathies' are said to be compounded into what is called Eclectic, which is therefore the most comprehensive of them, and at the same time the least original. Most other fallacies spring up at once," added the *Reporter*, "create a great sensation and often stagger and stun the intelligent, by the startling novelty of their propositions, bewilder the unwary by the immensity of their premises, and then die out. But the Eclectics keep themselves alive by swallowing everything which happens to turn up, until they have become like Macbeth's caldron, an extraordinary conglomeration of such incompatibles as Injun doctoring, Dutch homeopathy, water cure, electropathy, physiomedicalism, etc."[11]

Actually, this was a sarcastic oversimplification of the basic tenets of the sect. True, the eclectics were open to almost any medical theory of the day, but they did not shun formal education like the early Thomsonians. Beach established the first sectarian college in the United States with his Reformed Medical College of the City of New York in 1830, then later moved his facility to Ohio under the name Worthington Medical College, which opened in the winter that same year.[12] The Worthington school had a difficult time, however. Poor organization, low enrollment, faculty dissension, and accusations of grave robbing to fill dissection needs all spelled disaster for the college. In 1840 the state of Ohio refused to renew its charter. Undaunted, Thomas Vaughan Morrow (1804–1850), who had been with Beach from the beginning, secured a charter from the state on March 10, 1845, to open a school under the name Eclectic Medical Institute of Cincinnati. Thus, Morrow became affectionately regarded as "the moving spirit of the college" and "the father of the Institute and of Eclecticism in the West."[13] Where the Worthington school faltered, the Eclectic Medical Institute (hereafter EMI) flourished. By the 1850s it had grown to become one of the largest medical schools in the country and graduated well over a quarter of all Ohio-educated practitioners in that decade.[14] For nearly a century, the EMI served as "the mecca of eclectic thinking" and "the mother institute of reformed medicine."[15] "The educated irregulars," observes Ronald L. Numbers, "particularly among the homeopaths and eclectics, simply were not the incompetent charlatans their enemies made them out to be."[16]

If the allopaths underrated the eclectics' devotion to education, they also unfairly characterized their therapeutics. The eclectics attacked the allopathic practices of bleeding and massive dosing with calomel and other minerals and adhered to a vegetable materia medica consisting mostly of plants indigenous to America. Casting the eclectics as little more than a collection of amorphous suffixes as the *Medical and Surgical Reporter* had done was unfair; the general emphasis of their therapeutics changed with time but was nonetheless discernible. Over the course of its century-long existence, eclectic therapeutics may be broadly divided into three periods: (1) from 1830 to 1850, the "antiphlogistic" years, a system of therapeutics aimed at contravention of fever and inflammation; (2) from 1850 to the Civil War, the age of the commercial concentrates (the resins, resinoids, alkaloids, and oleoresins); and (3) the era of "specific medication," from 1870 to the fading away of eclecticism itself in the 1930s and 1940s.[17] As can be seen from this periodization, the eclectics placed great store in their therapeutic agents.

Thus, in 1870 John Uri Lloyd stood on the brink of the last great phase of American eclecticism. King, who had been carefully watching the progress of Lloyd ever since his apprenticeship to Gordon, now asked the young pharmacist to examine and experiment with some of the "present formulae" of the eclectics. This was ostensibly to assist King in the preparation of an eclectic pharmacopeia sponsored by a number of state eclectic medical societies. In September of 1870, Lloyd was formally introduced to the eclectic world: "I have engaged," announced King, "a young man who is a talented and skillful pharmacist, Mr. J. U. Lloyd, now in Mr. O. F. Gordon's drugstore, to experiment with these unsatisfactory preparations, and ascertain what improvements can be made thereon. The results of his experiments will be published, from time to time, in the Eclectic Medical Journal. . . ."[18]

Early in 1871, King then suggested an even closer alliance with the eclectic cause, one with far-reaching implications for the young drug clerk. King offered Lloyd the opportunity of becoming the developer of a new American materia medica with H. M. Merrell. King explained both sides of the situation. On the one hand, by joining up with H. M. Merrell he would be allying himself with those outside the fold of regular practice. "As you know," admitted King to Lloyd, "the terms 'quack' and 'charlatan' are freely applied to us." On the other hand, Lloyd's acceptance would grant him access to "exceptional educational and research opportunities." King continued:

> Never did a young American pharmacist have such a chance as will finally come to you by the development of this new field, the American materia medica. In the professional phases of our crusade you need take no part, nor need you concern yourself in any way in our principles of medication. . . . All we ask is that you study the drugs of our materia medica and develop its pharmacy in such a way as to permit *all* physicians to practice with certainty, so far as our *medicines* are concerned. If you

authorize me to say that you are willing to consider this proposition, both Mr. Merrell and Dr. Scudder will talk it over with
you.[19]

King's discussion was not entirely candid, for there is no way that a drug
manufacturer or pharmaceutical chemist could develop the eclectic
pharmacy without himself becoming associated with eclecticism.

Lloyd was not the first one to produce eclectic preparations in the
Queen City. Indeed, precedents in that realm indicated success and prosperity: chief among them, William S. Merrell (1798–1880). He came
to Cincinnati in 1828, a college-educated chemist and former school-
teacher.[20] On June 10 of that year, Merrell made his very first drug sale
from his Western Market Drug Store. Merrell's reputation advanced in
the city, and late in 1846, a little more than a year after the chartering
of the EMI, he was asked to move his operations to the institute on the
corner of Court and Plum Streets to make the many botanical preparations that formed every eclectic physician's armamentarium. By so doing, Merrell attached himself to eclectic medicine for the remainder of
his life. It was a wise decision, for he prospered under the relationship
and became a powerful presence within the institute itself and within
eclecticism generally. From 1864 until his death some sixteen years later,
Merrell was president of the board of trustees for the EMI,[21] and he was
acknowledged by fellow eclectics as the "father" of their distinctive botanical pharmacy.[22] So why was John King skipping over this doyen of
eclectic medicines in favor of a relatively unknown and youthful clerk?

To answer this, we must go back to the second phase of eclectic
therapeutics: the concentrates. This line of pharmaceuticals was first discussed by King in 1846. "For the last several years," announced King,
"I have prepared my medicines, or rather those of which I make frequent use, in such a manner, that the doses, in quantity, are much smaller
than usual, and are fully as effectual in their results, if not more so, than
the same articles as generally administered."[23] Although he did not prepare each in the same way, his description of one class of preparations
would prove significant. "From some I obtain only the resins, by extracting all that Alcohol will take up, then filter the Alcoholic tincture,
to which [I] add an equal quantity of water, and separate the Alcohol
by distillation—the resin sinks to the bottom. . . . Sometimes I distil

[*sic*] the Alcoholic tincture to a certain quantity without the addition of water, and then evaporate the remainder, until the residue is of the required consistence for pilular extract, or powder. . . ." Thus King described, for the first time, the making of an eclectic concentrate. King's own vague words "from *some*" and "*sometimes*" demonstrate the unscientific and imprecise nature of these products. It is this lack of scientific rigor and systematic phytochemical study that, in the words of the leading historian of the botanico-medical movement, "doomed so much of eclectic pharmacy to scientific sterility and gross empiricism."[24]

Despite his founding role in this class of preparations, King did little to promote their widespread use; it was William S. Merrell who began marketing the eclectic concentrations commercially in 1847. Admitting a lack serious chemical analysis in their manufacture, Merrell declared: "Our efforts are directed, not to the improvement of Chemistry but of Medicine; not to make scientific analyses of plants, but to present their medicinal principles in a concentrated, definite, and economical form, as articles of the Materia Medica."[25] The nomenclature employed in promoting Merrell's concentrates reveal much. Merrell applied the generic *in* suffix to natural substances like podophyllum (sold as podophyllin) and even generalized these nonvolatile, solid or semisolid plant exudations not as resins but as resinoid (resinlike), making his medicines of uncertain and indefinite strength and efficacy. In short, with vague generic names concocted out of inexact formulas, the most precise thing about them was that they were concentrates—exactly *of what* and *what from* was arbitrary and unclear.

Nevertheless, these eclectic concentrations elicited considerable praise and sales. Some of the EMI faculty were swept away by these products. Professor of materia medica, therapeutics, and medical botany G. W. L. Bickley (1823–1867) called them "most beautiful preparations;"[26] Robert S. Newton (1818–1881), the editor of the *Eclectic Medical Journal*, exclaimed, "The great convenience of this form of remedies, to say nothing about the benefit to the patient, is incalculable;"[27] and adjunct professor of pathology Walter Miller Ingalls pronounced the concentrates the harbinger of "a better day coming for the Eclectic practice of medicine."[28] With such a receptive market, others quickly followed in Merrell's wake to produce similar concentrated medicines. One of the leaders was B. Keith and Company, but others included F. D. Hill of

Cincinnati, T. C. Thorp of Cincinnati, Tilden and Company of New York, and William H. Baker and Company of St. Louis.

Others were less enthusiastic. William Procter Jr., an important and influential pharmacist of the day, had already expressed doubts about the botanico-medical movement in general in 1854, referring to eclecticism as "a *scheme* [emphasis added] of medicine and pharmacy."[29] Now he voiced serious concerns over the concentrated medicines of B. Keith and Company. In 1855 a three-hundred-page book titled *Positive Medical Agents*, published "by authority of the American Chemical Institute" (i.e., B. Keith and Company), was released, billing itself as "a treatise on the new alkaloid, resinoid, and concentrated preparations of indigenous and foreign medical plants."[30] Procter correctly observed that, deceptively disguised as a serious scholarly production, the real purpose of the book was to promote Keith's line of products.

Some eclectics were worried about this concentration craze as well. Since 1855 John King had expressed his concern for the purity of these concentrated medicines. Pointing to the B. Keith company as one selling "Pure Concentrated Medicines" that were adulterated, King warned of the harm these poor preparations could do to the eclectic cause: "Already are the old-school [allopathic] physicians manifesting an interest in our concentrated remedies," he warned, "and if we permit such trash to be foisted on them as pure agents, they will believe that Eclecticism is indeed quackery and humbug, and it will require years to overcome the effects of such a disgraceful blow."[31]

Statements like this intensified already strained relations within the EMI and the professional fold. During this time the eclectic ranks broke into civil war over a variety of causes, not the least of which involved arrangements between Robert S. Newton and B. Keith and Company to publish an *American Eclectic Dispensatory* that would actively promote the concentrated medicines and thus form a rival to King's *American Dispensatory* (the eclectic equivalent to the *United States Dispensatory*). This led John King, Joseph R. Buchanan, Ichabod G. Jones, William Sherwood, John Wesley Hoyt, and Charles Harley Cleaveland to form a new Eclectic College of Medicine.[32] Thus, while the *Eclectic Medical Journal* heaped glowing adjectives upon Merrell's and others' concentrated "remedies," other journals, including the opposing faction's *College Journal of Medical Science*, voiced serious doubts about pursuing the marketing

of more and more concentrated products with reckless abandon. A professor of chemistry at the allopathic Ohio Medical College, Edwin S.
Wayne (1818–1885), published a four-page critique of the concentrations made by B. Keith and Company in the *American Journal of Phar-*
macy. Not surprisingly, Wayne found another ready outlet for his scrutiny
of the concentrates in the *College Journal*:

> This class of medicines, it is true, have met with much fa-
> vor, and the pharmaceutists who are engaged in the preparation
> of them, are adding from time to time to the list, seemingly
> satisfied that if they can obtain a resin, or precipitate, by the
> simple process mentioned, that they have obtained the active
> principles of the substance thus treated.
>
> These resins as mentioned, are said to be the active principle
> of vegetable substances, and as such appear to be acknowledged
> by common consent, without any attempt to investigate the
> subject. This is a point that demands some further examination;
> and it will be found, upon examination, to be an assertion only,
> and with but little fact to base it on.
>
> To show that these resins, and oleo-resins [i.e., an oil hold-
> ing resin in solution, extracted by means of alcohol], are not in
> all instances the active, or medicinal properties of plants in a
> concentrated form, is the object I have in view in writing this
> article; and also, to induce the medical faculty to investigate this
> matter a little more attentively than they have done, so as not
> to be deceived into the use of substances possessing little or
> none of the active principle of the plant or root that it repre-
> sents.[33]

Wayne's assessment was objective and accurate, and the *College Jour-*
nal allowed William S. Merrell the opportunity to answer his pointed
review of the concentrates:

> Mr. W. certainly knows that the hydrastine and the sangui-
> narina, prepared in this city, are precipitated by chemical
> reägents, from the "residuary water" after the subsidence of the
> resins. Of the articles which I have introduced scarcely any two

are prepared by just the same process. It is true that the first steps in the process are generally the same. The substance operated on is in most cases first exhausted by alcohol, either pure or a little diluted; for we hold that all the medicinal or poisonous elements of every organic substance *while in their natural combinations* are soluble in that menstruum, while for the most part the inert and simply nutritive elements are not soluble in it. Here we employ this important but expensive agent, to separate them, and having thus far isolated the medicinal elements of a plant, we then concentrate them with suitable modifications, to a certain standard, and call the preparation a *fluid extract*, or to the pilular consistence, and name it an *alcoholic extract* . . . and put them up under such names we think appropriate. And in no case have we "taken it for granted," that a precipitate which we have obtained, whether by water only or by chemical reägents, is as such (unless where its sensible qualities are sufficient evidence), until experiment in its use has demonstrated that it is so.

So far, therefore, as our establishment is concerned, or that of others of the more respectable manufacturers of these medicines, the above article has no application.[34]

Merrell's response to Wayne was evasive. Admitting that "scarcely any two are prepared by just the same method," Merrell failed to explain exactly what those methods were. Merrell did not even hint at what he meant by concentrating "with suitable modifications" made to "a certain standard." What modifications? What standard? Although Merrell claimed to have submitted his concentrates to experimental analysis, he offered no concrete example of having done so. Furthermore, Merrell offered no clear and consistent principles dictating the naming of his products, only referring vaguely to marketing them "under such names we think appropriate." Taken in its entirety, Merrell's reply merely substantiated many of Wayne's charges.

As mentioned earlier, John King, despite his introduction of the concentrating process, remained wary of many of the commercial usages of these products. Objecting to the vague terminology being used by Merrell and other commercial manufacturers, King declared, "I now wish to call the attention of all classes of physicians to a most stupendous fraud which is being perpetrated upon them in relation to concentrated preparations in which oils, oleo-resins, fluid extracts, etc., are triturated with finely powdered *green* leaves, or roots, or barks, perhaps of the crude articles of which they purport to be concentrations, as well as with rosin, carbonate of magnesia, etc. The resin of jalap, which can be obtained for two dollars a pound, is triturated with some inert agent, and sold for Jalapin at one dollar an ounce; and similar impositions."[35]

Lloyd himself noted that King's usage of concentrates was much more restrained compared with the haphazard applications of the commercial manufacturers. "Be it observed that these concentrated principles were by Dr. King called *dried hydro-alcoholic extracts*," he pointed out, "and also that the list does not include any drug dominated by a poisonous or active resin or oleo-resin. Notwithstanding criticisms and unfounded statements to the contrary, it is seen that, at that early date, the very opening of the American Materia Medica, Dr. King had instituted an intelligent classification of these substances that should not have been neglected." Lloyd added that under King's system "no blanket title would have been necessary. Had it been adopted, the so-called alkaloids, concentrations, or resinoids, that plagued Eclectic pharmacy in succeeding years, would have been unknown."[36] Lloyd is perhaps too optimistic here and hangs excessive importance upon the descriptive nomenclature employed in promoting this line of botanicals, but there is no doubt that poor and imprecise terminology lent itself to a barrage of concentrated products of uncertain composition, strength, and purity sold on the open market. King had been opposed to manufacturers playing fast and loose with product names, particularly Merrell and Company.

All of this caused serious acrimony between Merrell and King. In an especially acerbic article, King responded to Merrell's charge that he had, among other things, represented the compound syrup of stillingia in his *Dispensatory* as an officinal "without giving us any credit for its origin. To this King answered that "he [Merrell] never gave me the formula," and went on to accuse Merrell of "nostrum mongering." Suggesting that physicians were being led more by the pecuniary designs of druggists rather than the true efficacy of any given medicine and that he would lead the fight against this growing problem, King added that "if Mr. Merrell, or others, are not disposed to aid in this laudable undertaking, preferring secrecy and individual interest to open, candid, scientific expositions for the benefit of medical science and humanity, he as well as they, must expect to be dropped along the highway."[37]

William S. Merrell was hardly one to be "dropped" even at the suggestion of so important an eclectic figure as Dr. John King; but the vicious infighting *was* dropped by 1859. Both parties realized that eclecticism had trouble enough without fighting their own civil war, and most of the rebel faculty returned to the EMI. While open wounds were healed, scars remained. In all early editions of King's *American Dispensatory*, the author acknowledged the assistance of William S. Merrell; but more revealingly he singled out Edwin S. Wayne, the outspoken critic of the eclectic concentrations, for special praise and thanks: "The latter gentleman [Wayne] ranks among the best practical and theoretical Chemists in our country."[38] Merrell and King might work together, but their relationship would remain cool and distant for the remainder of their lives. The problem was not that Merrell continued to manufacture eclectic concentrates. Practically all the eclectic drug houses marketed some concentrated medicines. Even Lloyd Brothers as late as 1910 offered an array of these products because they were "still desired by some physicians who read after the old authors," although they followed their price list of "Concentrations. Including 'Resinoids,' Alkaloids, Alkaloidal Salts, etc." with lengthy disclaimers as to the value and efficacy of the items offered therein.[39] The problem was Merrell's preeminent role in introducing this line of products commercially, his loose classification of product names in marketing them, and his vigorous defense of the flagrant and extreme empiricism employed in their development. In short, Merrell was simply too closely identified with a product line that "did not represent the therapeutic qualities of the structure from which it was derived."[40]

It is in this context that John King's offer to a youthful John Uri Lloyd barely in his twenties must be understood. A new man unaffiliated with any of the previous nostrums was needed to research and develop a new line of medicines that would be promoted by King and Scudder. Because of Lloyd's collaboration with the Harlow M. Merrell firm (William S. Merrell's nephew, who had left his uncle's business to strike out on his own), specific medicines would not only be associated with a bright, young pharmaceutical researcher but also with a known rival to the William S. Merrell Company. King made himself perfectly clear on the matter: "The trash on the market, under the free-to-all name of 'fluid extracts,' illustrates that, for protection, our preparations must be distributed under protected labels. . . . Furthermore," he added, "we must resist not only the shot-gun approach heired by our neighbors, the old school, but we must soften the processes and modify the opinions of old-time Eclectics. We will surely offend all pharmacists engaged in making and marketing the old-style conglomerates, for their syrups, elixirs and fluid extracts are crudities that must also surely become obsolete. Our aim is to introduce and employ exact representatives of fresh vegetable drugs, free from inert constituents, supplied under their true botanical names."[41]

These new medications were not really King's at all but rather the work of John Milton Scudder (1829–1894). Scudder's ideas of "specifics" related to a broad conceptual framework that included disease, disease "expression," and diagnosis.[42] Scudder's most significant contribution, however, came with his ideas of specific medications, first introduced in the pages of the *Eclectic Medical Journal* in 1869. Scudder's book-length work that appeared the following year announced what would become the defining therapeutics of American eclecticism during the last third of its existence: a system of specific medication tied directly to a system of specific diagnosis.[43] Moreover, it was in the *preparation* of specific medicines that the departure from previous practice could be seen:

> I insist that all vegetable remedies should be prepared from the *recent* crude material obtained at its proper season. In some cases the remedy does not materially deteriorate within the year, and may be kept in stock until the next season for gathering. But in all cases it is better if prepared at once after gathering, and in many the preparation should be from the *fresh* article before any desiccation. The reasons are obvious—the medicinal properties are found in the juices of the plant, or stored in its cells, principally of the bark. In both cases drying removes the medicinal principle, to a greater or lesser extent. The medicinal principles of plants are to a considerable extent

complex and unstable organic bodies, and time, with its constant processes of change and decay, changes, deteriorates, and finally destroys them.[44]

In some senses, there was not anything truly new here. Many of Scudder's ideas were derived from the homeopaths and even the physio-medicals. But being admittedly eclectic in using remedies was no disgrace. Even years after the introduction of Scudder's Specifics, Lloyd reminded the dispensing pharmacist that "several of the Specific Medicines are representatives of drugs originally introduced by the Homeopathic profession, who should be given the credit due them. Aconite, Pulsatilla, Bryonia, Staphisagria are examples."[45]

Whatever the originality of these first specifics, Scudder and King needed a bright and ambitious person in the research and development of more varieties of these medicines exclusively for their products. King and Scudder wanted to protect these new "specific medicines" from a repetition of the eclectic concentrations debacle. "To prevent the fraudulent imitations that will surely follow unless we safeguard them," warned Scudder, "they are to be protected under a characteristic label. This label I have already devised, copyrighted and given the rights of use to H. M. Merrell."[46] King and Scudder's concerns about distributing these specific medicines under "protected labels" were not unfounded. Almost immediately following Scudder's initial discussion of his specifics, several of Cincinnati's drug manufacturers began advertising "Specific Medicines." This occurred until copyright had been secured and exclusive rights conveyed to H. M. Merrell.[47] Unlike the earlier eclectic concentrations, Scudder's Specific Medicines could now be manufactured and distributed by H. M. Merrell and himself only.

But what was in it for young John Uri Lloyd? Actually, the eclectic cause presented several compelling advantages. First, the explanation of the situation made it clear that Scudder wanted *only* H. M. Merrell to produce his Specifics, thus placing Lloyd in the enviable position of being the exclusive pharmaceutical chemist working on formulating this class of products. Second, he would be working with a man who had been located at the EMI building since 1861, successor to the well-known T. C. Thorp establishment, who in turn had succeeded William S. Merrell at the EMI headquarters in 1854. By the time of King's offer for Lloyd to join the Merrell firm, H. M. Merrell (with Thorp as a secondary partner) had been running an established, respected pharmaceutical house for a decade. Third, all the advantages that King had outlined were true: Lloyd would have access to outstanding research facilities, and the prospect of being the exclusive producer of a fresh and systematically developed class of medicines was tantalizing. Fourth, by allying himself with the eclectics, he would have a large and ready market for his products. Although not the largest sectarian group nationally and far smaller than the allopaths everywhere, the eclectics outnumbered all other "irregulars" in Ohio, Indiana, and Illinois.[48] Besides this, a close connection to eclecticism was not tantamount to an end of one's professional standing and respectability. Of all the botanico-medical groups, it was the eclectic faction which attracted the "more able and better educated men."[49] The prospects of this association for a man so young and comparatively inexperienced were undeniably alluring. Lloyd answered King's proposition with an unequivocal "yes."

Despite Lloyd's persistent complaints of being ostracized for his decision to join King and Scudder, he admitted that "the majority of my friends in 'old school' circles stood by me faithfully."[50] A few valued colleagues, however, namely Lloyd's old professor of chemistry, Roberts Bartholow, and the prominent Cincinnati chemist, Edwin S. Wayne, held nothing against Lloyd personally but felt that he was damaging his career and future opportunities.

Despite the concerns of Bartholow and Wayne, the close connection of Lloyd with Scudder and King placed him in the inner sanctum of eclecticism: King and Scudder were the unrivaled driving forces within the institute and throughout the movement nationally.[51] Scudder had considerable business acumen. In the wake of the eclectic concentrate craze and the EMI schism of the 1850s, Scudder took charge of the school in 1862 and systematically went about the work of restoring its academic and financial integrity. His prolific pen and editorial work for the *Eclectic Medical Journal* from 1862 until his death in 1894 made him, in Otto Juettner's words, "the great exponent of the tenets of therapeutic faith adhered to and believed by the Eclectic school. In fact, *he was the Eclectic school*, because every phase of its life bore the impress of his powerful individuality."[52] King's influence in the eclectic movement was equally impressive. Fluent in French and German, King was a talented and urbane man whose forty-two years of teaching obstetrics made him an awe-inspiring role model for his students. He was so inextricably associated with his monumental *American Dispensatory* that most eclectics referred to this pharmaceutical bible simply as "*King's Dispensatory.*" King was active and prominent in eclectic organizations at both the state and national levels. By the time of his death in 1893, his name was virtually synonymous with eclecticism. Lloyd always fondly remembered King's daily visits to Gordon's drugstore and his "fatherly interest" in his work.[53]

Lloyd's years from 1870 through early 1877 were filled with quiet study and hard work punctuated by opportunity, love, tragedy, and loss. As John King had promised in the September 1870 issue of the *Eclectic Medical Journal,* Lloyd reported the results of his investigations to his eclectic colleagues. From 1870 through 1876, he published fourteen articles on phytochemical and phytopharmaceutical topics.[54] Meanwhile, Nelson Ashley Lloyd was working as a drug clerk for H. Swannell in Champaign, Illinois, though his true desire was to remain in Cincinnati and work with his brother. In 1876 John and Ashley felt they had enough capital to realize their dream of working together. Returning to Cincinnati, Ashley joined John and rented a modest facility at 35-37 Canal Street. John resigned his position at H. M. Merrell's and commenced operations with his brother in November. Merrell and his partner T. C. Thorp, well aware of the seriousness of their loss, made John an attractive offer: They would offer to buy out all of Lloyd Brothers' stock, use half of the total to make the first payment on the purchase of Thorp's interest in Merrell's firm, and over a period of ten years Lloyd would take over Thorp's interest in the laboratory. T. C. Thorp would retain an active interest in the company as business manager, with his son Abner assuming the duties of bookkeeper. As of January 1877, the company's new name would be Merrell, Thorp, and Lloyd. Thus, almost as soon as it started, Lloyd Brothers again aborted operations, this time at least under considerably more favorable circumstances.[55] Ashley was out, but he found a Cincinnati-based job as salesman for Reakert, Hale, and Company, a local drug wholesaler.

At this same time, Lloyd's private life was also looking bright. While attending the Ninth Street Central Christian Church, he had met a young school teacher named Adeline Meader. Just twenty-one, the brown-haired, gray-eyed beauty swept Lloyd off his feet. They were married on December 27, 1876, when everything looked full of promise for the young pair: "Addie" loved her teaching at the Sixteenth District public school; Lloyd was about to enter into partnership with a respected and profitable drug wholesaler; and his brother was in town, doing well at Reakert, Hale, and Company. As part of their honeymoon, they journeyed to upstate New York to visit Lloyd's relatives. While on the train, Addie became seriously ill. On January 7, 1877, Lloyd's bride of eleven days died of acute peritonitis.[56]

John was understandably bereaved, but he was not crushed. He would eventually remarry. In 1880 he married Emma Rouse, the daughter of Thomas Rouse, patriarch of an old and venerable family from Boone and Grant Counties in Kentucky. She remained by John Uri's side for the next fifty-two years until her death in 1932, and together they raised three children: John Thomas, born in 1884; Anna, born in 1886; and Dorothy, born in 1894.

In the meantime, however, the driving ambition that impelled Lloyd forward sustained him during the difficult period following the death of Addie. John Uri Lloyd was a man whose mind was never far from business. The young pharmacist demonstrated early on a tenacity and perseverance in the face of difficulties that would have destroyed many men. Lloyd found solace in two great healers: time and work. Brighter days were surely ahead.

4

Busy with Business:
From Merrell, Thorp, and Lloyd
to Lloyd Brothers

Early records give every indication that if young John Uri Lloyd was anything he was *ambitious*. Lloyd's connection with the powerful figures of King and Scudder opened the door to numerous professional contacts, and his correspondence shows a careful cultivation of associations and friendships with prominent individuals in the medical profession. Names like Roberts Bartholow (1831–1904), the famous Cincinnati physician, Charles Rice (1841–1901), the important pharmacist at New York's Bellevue Hospital, John M. Maisch (1831–1893), the editor of the *American Journal of Pharmacy* and first permanent secretary of the American Pharmaceutical Association, and Edward R. Squibb (1819–1900), a physician and pioneer pharmaceutical manufacturer, grace the extant archival files of Lloyd's correspondence. These letters, written during Lloyd's first business partnership with Merrell and Thorp in 1877 up to the emergence of an independent Lloyd Brothers manufacturing concern in 1885, are clearly the work of an ambitious young man very busy with business.[1] It could be that he was working to forget the tragic loss of his young bride Addie, but even as an apprentice, Lloyd expressed to family members his desire to "get rich."[2]

This frank admission was in keeping with the times. Social Darwinism, the reigning zeitgeist of the Gilded Age, equated wealth with worth as part of a natural selection theory that had gained widespread popularity following the Civil War. Americans had adopted a business ideology of classical liberalism that put tremendous faith in a laissez-faire economy. This financial free-for-all was justified by social theorists such as Herbert Spencer in England and Charles Graham Sumner in the United States who elevated the resulting inequities of the haves and have-nots to supposedly inexorable "laws of nature." Whatever the modern reader may think of this prescription for unbridled rapacity in the public sector, such attitudes were not only common but praised in a period that saw financial success as an expression of divine sanction contributing to the national destiny. "Because of the heroic role of business in the post Civil War era," writes historian Alfred Thimm, "this business ideology was widely adopted by the American public; and until the Great Depression at least, the vulgarized dogma of classical liberalism have been an integral part of American folklore."[3] It is important to understand from the outset that Lloyd was both influenced by and reflective of this business ethos. After all, this was, according to Thimm, the "secular religion of the bourgeoisie."[4] It is in this context that we see a young, eager, and ambitious John Lloyd working toward establishing his own drug manufacturing concern.

Lloyd could not have been laboring in a more favorable economic climate. While it is true that the years 1873 through 1896 have been generally described by economic historians as a "long-wave" depression in which overall price levels declined nearly ten points (e.g., 56.6 in 1885 to 46.5 in 1896), this period was also marked by energetic investment, strong business upswings, and vast expansion of the manufacturing sector.[5] Concomitantly, there was a permanent shift away from a rural, agrarian society to an urban, industrial one: farmworkers represented 58.9 percent of the labor force in 1860, but by century's end made up a mere 37.5 percent of all workers.[6] America was changing.

These kinds of fundamental economic transformations propelled large-scale drug manufacturing forward. The specific driving forces at work enlarging the structure and scope of the drug industry manifested primarily in two broad areas. First were the scientific advances that coincided with the development of an industrial infrastructure to allow—even mandate—a more modernized pharmaceutical manufacturing. In the early nineteenth century, investigations by German and French pharmacists and chemists established the principles whereby alkaloids (bitter tasting, alcohol-soluble organic compounds of vegetable origin), glycosides (a group of compounds that yield a sugar and an alcohol or phenol when hydrolized), and halogens (the chlorines, iodines, and bromines finding therapeutic uses in the mid- to late nineteenth century) could be uniformly produced to create mass-marketed medicines. Indeed, these processes required procedures and equipment not available to the individual pharmacist. For the development of medicinal plant products, the alkaloid and glycoside extraction techniques in particular were heralding a new pharmaceutical era. "The availability of the active principle," write two noted authorities, "now concentrated as a chemical rather than dispersed throughout a crude drug, meant that purity, strength, standardization, and dosage could be controlled as never before."[7] The *USP* reflected these changes in the growth of official fluidextracts that were rapidly replacing the cruder oils and tinctures of an earlier era. The *USP* of 1890, for example, retained almost one-third of the items of the 1820 edition, but by the eighth revision in 1900, many of the older botanical drugs were dropped in favor of mass-produced fluidextracts; the *USP* of 1900 listed eighty-five fluidextracts of vegetable drugs.[8] These shifts brought about by significant scientific innovations led to a decline in the individual art of the apothecary in the nineteenth century in favor of medicines manufactured to standards of unprecedented uniformity and quality.

These changes can be seen most clearly in the kinds of pharmaceutical preparations common to the industry in the 1880s. To begin, there were two broad categories of pharmaceuticals: liquids and solids. Basically, there were two types of "officinals" (i.e., preparations listed in the pharmacopeia and expected to be kept on hand at any fully equipped apothecary): those preparations made by extracting the soluble principles of a crude drug by passing a suitable solvent through it (known as percolation or displacement), and those made without this process. Either type could be a solid or a liquid. Of the solids, those made by percolation were the extracts, abstracts, and resins; those made without this process were powders, triturations, masses, confections, pills, troches, cerates, ointments, plasters, papers, and suppositories. By far, the most extensive group of preparations was the liquids; they too could be made with or without percolation. Examples of the former were the infusions and decoctions comprising the aqueous liquids (infusions, i.e., vegetable substances treated with hot or cold water, and decoctions, i.e., vegetable substances boiled in water), alcoholic liquids (tinctures, wines, and fluidextracts), ethereal liquids (oleoresins, i.e., the oils and resins extracted from plants by percolation with ether), and the acetous liquids (vinegars of lobelia, opium, sanguinaria, and squill); examples of those officinal liquids made without percolation were the aqueous solutions (the so-called waters and solutions), the aqueous solutions containing sweet, glutinous or sticky substances (syrups, honeys, mucilages, mixtures, and glycerites), the alcoholic solutions (spirits and elixirs), the ether solutions of the topical collodions (collodium, collodium cum cantharide, collodium flexile, and collodium stypticum), and the oil and fatty oil solutions (liniments and oleates).[9] Of all these preparations, the fluidextracts were having the greatest impact. As Joseph Remington in 1885 explained:

> Fluid extracts were officinal for the first time in 1850, and the list was then made up of *seven* concentrated preparations, although but *one* of these could be called a fluid extract within the present meaning of the term; of the seven, two were oleoresins, four were concentrated syrups, and but one a concentrated tincture. Since 1850 the use of fluid extracts has increased to an enormous extent, and the Pharmacopoeia of 1880 contains formulas for *seventy-nine*, the list embracing a greater number than any other class of preparations in the work. Fluid extracts may be justly called, "American preparations," and the advance made in pharmacy in this country within the last quarter of a century is largely due to the stimulus given to the studies in percolation by the demand for these useful liquids.[10]

Remington suggested that the reasons for the popularity of the fluidextracts was in their shelf life, their uniformity, and their concentration. This last feature should not be equated with the eclectic concentrations of the William S. Merrell and B. Keith firms and others, which were largely hodgepodge concoctions of green extracts. These mass-produced fluidextracts were inundating the drug market.

The second broad manifestation of large-scale drug manufacturing was taking place in the pharmaceutical houses themselves. Merrell, Thorp, and Lloyd was not the only one actively engaged in producing botanical medicines. By 1877, the year that Lloyd joined Merrell and Thorp, there were a number of comparatively large botanical drug companies operating in the United States. Besides Merrell and Company and B. Keith and Company, there were other specialists in botanical drugs, including Tilden and Company, a firm based in New Lebanon, New York, dating back to 1847; H. H. Hill and Company of Cincinnati; and one of the leaders in the field, H. Hillier's Sons Corporation of New York City. While chemical drugs were a growing commodity on the pharmacist's shelves, nearly all pharmaceutical firms in the United States carried a considerable stock of phytomedicinal products up until World War I: Smith Kline and French of Philadelphia and Parke Davis and Company of Detroit were large pharmaceutical manufacturers with a particularly extensive array of botanicals. The chemotherapies and the synthesis of organic chemicals that occurred during the last quarter of the nineteenth century was the domain of German research and development up until that time. A company like Mallinckrodt of St. Louis that focused its work on "pure chemicals for use in medicine" was the exception to the rule. Most manufacturers' product lines consisted of medicaments derived from an extensive and well-established vegetable materia medica.[11] Although botanical drugs would eventually be supplanted by chemical synthetics and biologicals (e.g., vaccines, antitoxins, and serums), Charles L. Huisking, who entered the drug trade at thirteen in 1898 and reminisced about the vast changes in the industry seventy years later, made the revealing observation that, practically speaking, when he started in the business "*drug* meant any product of the vegetable kingdom that was not chiefly used as food. . . . " "The crude trade was exceedingly complex," he added, "[representing] over 11,500 items, many of them in several distinct grades or varieties." He further noted that the highly variable nature of quality, supply, and demand for thousands of medicinal plant products made the market "no place for an ignorant or unwary operator."[12] In short, the well-known botanicals were no longer the exclusive domain of the compounding pharmacist but were being subjected to manufacture on an unprecedented scale.

Another important component of the drug industry in the late nineteenth century was the tremendous rise in proprietary medicines. This was a period that still saw most Americans using home remedies as the first line of defense against illness. These *patent* medicines (i.e., products prepared from secret formulas for direct consumer sale, distinguished by their use of trademarked names that bestowed proprietary rights to the owners) should be distinguished from *patented* medicines, which by definition means medicines whose formulas are given full disclosure. The producers of proprietary or patent medicines were utilizing mass-marketing techniques in newspapers and popular magazines to saturate the public with a variety of nostrums more noted for their descriptive innovations than their diagnostic accuracy. Unlike the so-called ethical drugs sold through a physician's prescription or exclusively for a physician's use in compounding his own preparations (often referred to during the period as "office pharmacy"), these concoctions were retailed over the counter to cure everything from a simple headache to less definable illnesses such as "torpid liver," "female complaint," "nervous prostration," "brain fatigue," "general debility," and "bad blood." While not all were botanically based, many such as Lydia Pinkham's Vegetable Compound, Morison's Pills, Godfrey's Cordial, Bateman's Drops, Mrs. Winslow's Soothing Syrup, and Kopp's Baby's Friend, were.[13] In 1880 there were 2,700 proprietary cure-alls on the market; by 1916 this class of remedy expanded to 38,000 items, fourteen times that of thirty years earlier.[14]

In 1877 the new partner in Merrell, Thorp, and Lloyd faced some formidable tasks: He would have to develop a new line of ethical drugs in a pharmaceutical environment already inundated with botanical products. He would also have to compete with the proprietary medicines capturing an ever larger market share. And above all, he would have to win over the vast majority of eclectic physicians by capitalizing on the very thing that made his Specific Medicine distinctive, its direct link to Scudder's therapeutic and diagnostic system. Conversely, he was limited to eclectic physicians committed to Scudder's system; although specific medication captured most of their hearts and minds, the most recent historian of these sectarians has noted that "it could not be categorized as a universal practice among eclectics."[15]

Nevertheless, one year after joining with the firm as partner, Lloyd appears to have appreciably expanded the company's product line. In January of 1878, Merrell, Thorp, and Lloyd added 13 "new remedies" to its price list of 176 fluidextracts, 83 Specifics, and 14 miscellaneous preparations.[16] The firm's description of these products helps to clarify the distinctions of Specific Medicines apart from the other fluidextracts. Carefully adhering to Scudder's principles of obtaining essential ingredients from "*recent* crude material obtained at its proper season," the company processed these vegetable products into a highly concentrated alcoholic Specific consisting of sixteen troy ounces (7,680 grains) of "crude material" to sixteen fluid ounces of tincture.[17] Merrell, Thorp, and Lloyd went on to explain that their Specific Medicines were designed for the physician to carry out his "office pharmacy"; all the good doctor need do was dilute these "easily carried and dispensed" remedies to the recommended strength. In contrast, the fluidextracts were made from *dried material* in a hydroalcoholic or absolute alcoholic base. This, according to Lloyd, made the fluidextracts "differ in appearance, and in therapeutical action, from our 'Specific Medicines,' but we warrant them equal to any fluid extract upon the market." Perhaps. But Parke Davis and Company, a true American giant in this product line, listed 10 percent of their 353 fluidextracts as having met *USP*-approved standards.[18] By comparison, Merrell, Thorp, and Lloyd listed only gentian as *USP* quality. This of course does not mean that Merrell, Thorp, and Lloyd's fluidextracts were substandard, only that the reader of the price list is left guessing as to the exact methods employed in each item's preparation or the standards of quality applied to any given product. Technical matters aside, Merrell and Thorp praised the work of their new partner, describing Lloyd as one "known by the excellence of his remedies, throughout the entire country" and "ever in the laboratory, experimenting and investigating." High praise for a twenty-eight-year-old pharmacist after only a single year's partnership.

Largely through Lloyd's diligence in the laboratory, the years from 1877 to 1881 saw Merrell, Thorp, and Lloyd prosper. Sometimes, however, success can breed dissension, for it became clear to both aging partners, T. C. Thorp and H. M. Merrell, that the flourishing business offered considerable promise to their respective sons. Abner Thorp, who had been working as the company bookkeeper with his father since Lloyd's entry as a partner four years earlier, was looking forward to a bright future with the rising firm. Thus, when H. M. Merrell proposed the entry of his only son, Frank, into the partnership, both Thorps and Lloyd objected. They argued that such an arrangement would have made the business top-heavy; the business could handle four partners, but not five.

T. C. Thorp became so incensed that he threatened to withdraw from the business entirely if Merrell's son joined the firm. Amid some enmity, H. M. Merrell left to start a drug business with his son. Ashley Lloyd, seeing his chance to finally join his brother, purchased Merrell's share of the company and entered as the new fourth partner; now it was T. C. and Abner Thorp, Ashley and John Uri Lloyd. T. C. Thorp then demanded that the Lloyds either buy or sell their share of the business, in an obvious effort to consolidate the Thorp family control of the company. After consulting with numerous area physicians about their plight, Ashley and John searched hastily for a bank loan. They finally received an eleventh-hour approval from the National Lafayette Bank, a situation undoubtedly brought about by Dr. Scudder and other physicians having offered the bank security on the loan. After this, there was little doubt that the Lloyd brothers had numerous friends in the city actively supporting their business interests in drug manufacturing. As of August of 1881, the company consisted of Abner Thorp, Nelson Ashley, and John Uri Lloyd: The firm of Thorp and Lloyd Brothers was established.

The newly restructured firm continued to grow. By 1884 Thorp and Lloyd Brothers was boasting a catalog expanded to "eighty pages of pharmaceuticals." In addition, it was offering an array of medical supplies and apparatus that included pocket medicine cases, buggy cases, saddle bags, obstetrical and dental cases, hypodermic syringes and needles, atomizers, crutches, abdominal supporters, and numerous other items.[19] Still located at Court and Plum Streets, the company proclaimed itself the "Physicians' Headquarters for Pure Medicines." Despite its diversified inventory, the mainstay of Thorp and Lloyd Brothers continued to be an ever-expanding variety of dosage forms. The firm offered sixteen different product lines: Specifics, fluidextracts, solid extracts, powdered solid extracts, elixirs, syrups, confections, tinctures, medicated wines, liquors, ointments, cerates, plasters, concentrated resins and alkaloids, sugar-coated pills and granules, and miscellaneous preparations. Its most promoted product, however, was always one thing: Specific Medicines. While the price lists would give the complete inventory, the partners chose to take full-page ads in the eclectic journals that extolled the virtues of their 176 Specific Medicines covering the vegetable kingdom from achillea to zingiber. Some of the more popular of these included Specific Podophyllum, prescribed as a cathartic and gastrointestinal stimulant, and Specific Sanguinaria, a treatment for a variety of digestive, respiratory, and circulatory ailments.

It is clear both from the expansion of its product lines and the diversification of dosage forms that Thorp and Lloyd Brothers was prospering. Much of this is undoubtedly due to the fact that John Lloyd's work and his products were already well known to the pharmaceutical profession. Lloyd himself had contributed to the published proceedings of the American Pharmaceutical Association (APhA) ever since he reported on hydrocyanic acid in 1875.[20] In 1878 Lloyd served on the Business Committee of the APhA, and he chaired the Committee on Papers and Queries from 1879 to 1885. Thorp and Lloyd Brothers also exhibited its products at the 1881 annual meeting of the APhA. "This display for completeness as a rare collection," observed the Committee on Exhibitions, "was of great interest to the student of pharmacy, and attracted much attention; among the lot we note alstonia constricta bark, the Australian fever tree, true damiana, eucalyptus globulus, frankenia grandifolia, rhamnus purshiana, criodictyon glutinosum, etc."[21]

This promotional activity by Thorp and Lloyd Brothers was necessary. Old animosities with William S. Merrell remained, and the Merrell Company had been sending out fliers to pharmacists openly attacking Specific Medicines. Referring to Scudder's work in developing this line of eclectic preparations and the Lloyd brothers' manufacture of them, Merrell asserted that "the whole scheme appears like an effort to obtain extra prices from their confiding customers." Deriding Scudder's efforts at providing legal protections for the name Specific Medicine, Merrell concluded that he "will not hesitate to take advantage of a copyrighted label to shield his errors."[22]

Professional rivalries and business competition aside, the question of the comparative quantity and quality of Thorp and Lloyd Brothers' preparations remains. Comparisons with the Lloyd specialty, "Specific Medicines," are difficult to make because of the unique nature of the products themselves; since these products are not recognized by the *USP*, there is no professional standard by which to judge them effectively. Fluidextracts, however, are another matter. If we wish to gain some idea of the quantity and quality of Thorp and Lloyd manufactures, their fluidextract line can be juxtaposed against a large and well-known pharmaceutical house already established in the botanical market. Again, as before, Parke Davis serves as a good benchmark. In 1885, for example, Parke Davis and Company made 494 fluidextracts (141 more than in 1879), while Thorp and Lloyd Brothers' output had skyrocketed from 176 different fluidextracts in 1878 to 835 by 1884. In just six years, Lloyd added 658 *new* fluidextracts to the company product line. Interestingly, Thorp and Lloyd Brothers assured their prospective customers that "the Pharmacopoeia of the United States, 1882 [the sixth decennial revision], is our authority *of all pharmaceuticals* [emphasis added] recognized by that work."[23] An item-by-item check against the *USP VI* reveals that this claim is not entirely correct. Of the 140 items listed as formulated according to *USP* standards, 5 fluidextracts made by Thorp and Lloyd Brothers are *not* designated as official ("*offi*") despite the fact that they are contained in the *USP*. Those items include cotton root, glycyrrhiza (licorice), sarsaparilla and sarsaparilla compound, and serpentaria (Virginia snake root).[24] In contrast, where possible, all of Parke Davis's fluidextracts complied with pharmacopeial standards. Still, it would be unfair to cast Thorp and Lloyd's products as substandard on the basis of five errant botanicals. John Uri's main interest was, after all, in Specifics, *not* the fluidextracts that he considered outmoded by Scudder's therapeutic innovations.

Taking Scudder's *Specific Medication and Specific Medicines* for his guide, Lloyd attempted to formulate products from recently acquired, fresh vegetable products in definite strengths. Earlier preparations (especially the eclectic concentrations discussed previously), Scudder noted, were not formulated in this manner: "Solid or fluid extracts are found of all degrees of strength, from the highest named in the pharmacopeia to nothing. In many cases they are prepared from old and worthless crude material, that has partly or wholly lost its medicinal properties, yet it is sold in the same packages and at the same prices, as if good."[25] Scudder's recommendations to physicians can be taken as Lloyd's own criteria of manufacture: "Prepare remedies from recent crude material, of full strength, without heat, and return every package that does not come up to the full standard of strength and excellence." Those standards of "strength and excellence" were largely designed by Scudder, and some, though by no means all, were listed in his book. While several methods of preparation are given for these Specifics, most begin with the phrase, "Prepare a tincture from the fresh . . ."

How then might a Specific Medicine be defined on the basis of its preparation? Were Specific Medicines merely old tinctures with a new name? Lloyd tried to disassociate his products from this compelling linkage. "Specific Medicines are not necessarily alcoholic," he insisted, "for a few of the list are definite chemicals, such as inorganic acids and salts, whilst some dry alkaloids of American drugs of established value are embraced in the list. Such as these are not *tinctures*. If drug strength and menstruum of the *official tinctures* be a standard for the definition *tincture*, then there is not a tincture in the entire Specific Medicine list, for all are much stronger than official tinctures."[26] Neither was the distinguishing feature of Specific Medicine to be found in its definite or exact strength. As Lloyd pointed out, "Honestly made U.S.P. fluid extracts are *definite*. Honestly made U.S.P. tinctures are *definite*. Homeopathic diluted tinctures are *definite*, but are none of the above J. M. Scudder's 'Specific Medicines,' although specifics if honestly prepared are *definite medicines*, and unless they are honestly made from prime materials, they are not definite in composition, and can not be 'specifics,' whatever label is upon the bottle."[27] Thus, all Specific Medicines were "definite" in strength but not all "definite" medicines were specific. In actuality, despite all of Lloyd's efforts to make his medicines appear radically new and distinctive, the inescapable fact is that the vast majority of Specific Medicines *were* tinctures. Excepting Sodium Sulphite, Sodium Phosphate, Carbo Veg., Carbolic Acid, and Hydrochloric Acid, nearly all labels indicate 240 to 480 grains per fluid ounce of absolute alcohol.[28]

Having set forth some of the difficulties in precisely describing Specific Medicines, a fairly accurate definition might be the following: Specific Medicines were, with a few exceptions, highly concentrated *unofficial* tinctures (approximately eight times the strength of most official tinctures) of plant constituents extracted either by maceration or percolation. In keeping with Scudder's preference for using "the *fresh* article before any desiccation,"[29] Lloyd too insisted that with few exceptions, "in general I find that tinctures made from fresh herbs, containing essential oils, give better satisfaction than when prepared from the dry. Also that many of our American roots, if only partially dried, furnish tinctures superior to either the perfectly dry or freshly dry."[30]

The tour de force of Thorp and Lloyd Brothers was in the successful

formulation and marketing of Specific Medicines; beginning in 1886,
these would be marketed under the name Lloyd Brothers. Abner Thorp
had been taking a back seat in operations for some time, for Ashley was
attending to more and more of the business functions while John kept
late hours in the laboratory. Late in 1885, the inevitable happened: Thorp
bowed out and the brothers took complete control of the firm. Through
King and Scudder's promotions, John Uri Lloyd's active professional life,
and his numerous publications, the Lloyd name became well known and
synonymous with Specific Medicines. The November issue of the *Eclectic
Medical Journal* carried the first Lloyd Brothers advertisement as follows:

> The patrons of the firm Thorp & Lloyd Brothers, and the
> medical profession generally, are respectfully invited to address
> their communications in accordance with the above new firm
> address. We take it for granted that the business and professional
> reputation of the present members of the firm over this country
> is such as to render an introduction unnecessary. . . .
> We make no pretensions to exclusive privileges or occult
> powers. We, in a business like manner only, shall from time to
> time bring forward the improvement in pharmacy opened up
> in our laboratory by a systematic research. Our aim shall be to
> excel, and we believe that by the skilled attention afforded by
> our long inquiry into the medical products of plants, we will
> be able to produce many preparations as yet unapproached.[31]

Now there was an opportunity to bring in their youngest brother,
Curtis Gates. Curtis had lived in Cincinnati ever since he roomed with
Ashley and John in 1877. He too had taken up pharmacy in a drugstore
on Ninth and Elm streets. Like his brothers, he passed the Examining
Board of Cincinnati and became a registered pharmacist. But Curtis
developed a strong interest in botany, and he pursued the field (in both
senses of the word) with a passion. Finding a position with the Standard
Printing Company for a time, he made numerous contacts with writers
from all over the world and became acquainted with several noted natu-
ralists. Curtis's love of botany would naturally complement an operation
devoted to medicinal plant preparations, and in January of 1886, John
and Ashley gave their brother one-third interest in Lloyd Brothers. In

exchange, all that Curtis needed to do was devote himself to identifying plants that might be put to pharmaceutical uses. Having assisted John with the botanical aspects of their *Drugs and Medicines of North America* (1884), Curtis continued with the responsibility of searching out new medicinal plants. For Curtis, this was a delightful extension of his labor of love. In his pursuit of ever more vegetable products, Curtis would become the most traveled of the Lloyd brothers.

For the next forty years, the "executive board" of the Lloyd Brothers firm was set: Curtis Gates would serve as field representative for the company, traveling in search of new medical plants and examining foreign supply sources; Nelson Ashley would be the business manager, handling every financial aspect of the manufacturing concern; and John Uri would be the undisputed head of the company, leading the research and development of their products and their promotion to the medical community. John Lloyd's role as a pharmaceutical manufacturer must be considered in context: his was a firm specializing in selling to a unique clientele. Furthermore, in maintaining Lloyd Brothers' links to the professional community of physicians, pharmacists, and scholars, it was John's responsibility to keep the company in the forefront of its field. Whatever might be said of the strengths or weaknesses of such an arrangement, there can be no doubt that it worked for quite a while; pharmacists were dispensing what in general they simply called Lloyd's Specifics well into the twentieth century. (For an interesting account of a practicing pharmacist's perspective on Specific Medicines, see appendix 1.)

This strong, family-based company was typical of drug manufacturers of the time. During the late nineteenth century, even the large pharmaceutical companies had a distinctly nepotistic leadership. Jonathan Liebenau has aptly characterized the structure of the drug industry at this time: "The typical structure of pharmaceutical companies, as with other manufacturing firms, consisted of direct family control over all aspects of production, marketing and sales. Family firms in Philadelphia in 1890 usually had a paternalistic head or a leadership of partners, many of them descendants of the founders. Wyeth and Sons, Powers and Weightman, Rosengarten and Sons, and Smith Kline, all had nonhierarchical structures in which family members controlled major operations using no middle management."[32] Soon all of this would change as more and more companies developed departments and divisions requiring middle management personnel; but companies like Lloyd Brothers could continue to operate with a minimal administrative and managerial cadre well into the twentieth century. The primary reason for this was their comparatively small size. As illustrated in table 1, Lloyd Brothers was not in the geographic center of pharmaceutical manufacturing. In fact, of ten cities showing major output in the so-called ethical drug market, Cincinnati was last in a quantitative ranking of firms and product values. Thus, John Lloyd's role as a pharmaceutical manufacturer was geared to a small, highly selective market. As one historian has observed of the smaller firms, "As long as they held at least one assured market they were able to survive competition from large manufacturers."[33] Of course, for Lloyd Brothers that "one assured market" was the eclectic physicians; and in developing and promoting his products, Lloyd made important contributions that transcended his firm's sectarian idiosyncrasies. Many of these contributions stemmed from professional and public activities both *in and out of* pharmacy that were rooted in his efforts to gain respect from the American intelligentsia.

Each aspect of John Uri Lloyd's career shows demonstrable efforts

Drug Manufacturers in Ten Selected Cities, 1890

City	Firms	Employees	Officers/Clerks	Workers	Product Values
Philadelphia	339	718	324	386	$1,275,629
New York	177	296	61	234	$1,116,334
St. Louis	130	230	117	113	$344,913
Brooklyn	90	248	119	129	$401,359
Chicago	65	137	59	78	$291,641
Minneapolis	42	90	54	36	$139,461
San Francisco	29	49	28	20	$88,532
Baltimore	8	26	7	19	$24,311
Cleveland	7	14	4	10	$23,391
Cincinnati	7	15	6	9	$19,726

Source: Compendium of the Eleventh Census, 1890, Part II (Washington, GPO, 1894).

to gain this respect in some detail. Lloyd adopted the persona of an intellectual; consequently, he was impelled to study, invent, collect books, teach, lecture, theorize, and write, all from a strong desire for acceptance within a community of scholars of which he desperately wanted to be a part. In his laboratory, his library, his classroom, his personal study, and his offices at Lloyd Brothers, Lloyd reflected the activities of a remarkably versatile man. Lloyd was a man of many parts, but it is important to remember that every facet of his versatility found its center in a phrase that has revealingly been applied to other botanical sectarians: "a striving for respectability."[34] His research, teaching, professional associations, and writings all emanated from, or were influenced in some way by, this powerful motivator. This deep-seated desire for respect and recognition had its advantages, but it also led to excesses and eccentricities, the distinctive features of which will become sharper as the story develops. For now, however, we will leave Lloyd Brothers with John, Ashley, and Curtis duly installed and working together as the new year opened in 1886.

The firm was now at full maturity. The company remained small but vibrant into the twentieth century, and John Fearn, an eclectic physician with a long-standing relationship with the Lloyd Brothers firm, has left posterity a vivid description of operations at the manufacturing plant in 1907 (see appendix 2). But a new wave of pharmaceuticals and their conglomerate manufacturers would increasingly cast their long shadows on the Cincinnati company. Those shadows would ultimately engulf the Specific Medicines and relegate them to the annals of history, but not until John Uri Lloyd had made a mark in every field he touched.

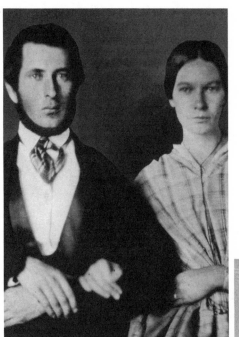

The parents of John Uri Lloyd (ca. 1848): Nelson Marvin and Sophia Webster Lloyd.

Young "Johnny," *left*, with brother Nelson Ashley and their mother Sophia (ca. 1853), about the time the Lloyds uprooted from upstate New York to live in northern Kentucky.

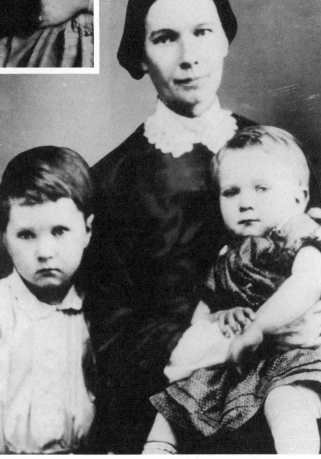

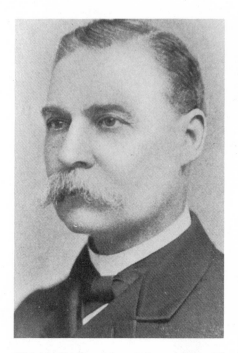
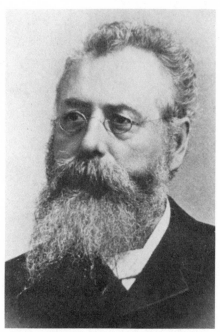

W. J. M. Gordon, *left*, and George Eger, Lloyd's instructors in the business and practice of pharmacy.

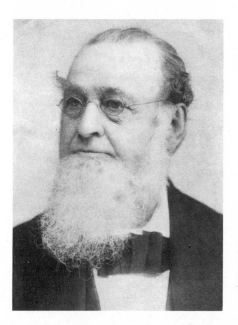
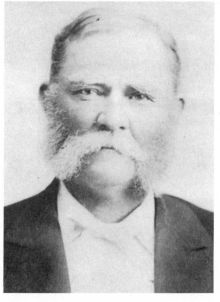

John King, *left*, and John Milton Scudder, leaders of eclecticism and Lloyd's mentors. During their lifetimes, King, Scudder, and Lloyd formed the brain trust of the eclectic medical movement in America.

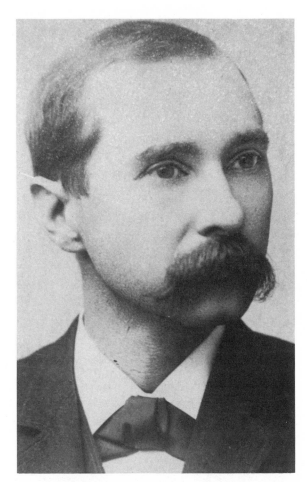

Lloyd as a young man
(ca. 1879).

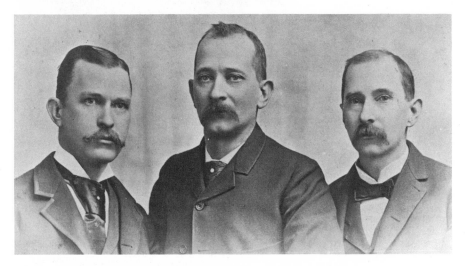

The Lloyd brothers (ca. 1879). *Left to right:* Curtis, Nelson, and John.

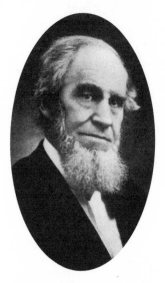

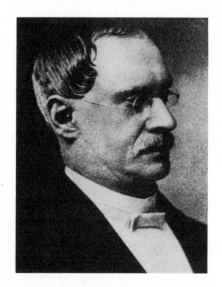

William S. Merrell, often referred to as the "father" of eclectic botanical medicines.

Charles Rice, Lloyd's confidant and long-standing friend. (Photo courtesy of the American Institute of the History of Pharmacy, Madison, Wisconsin)

This promotional pamphlet (ca. 1887) was one of the many marketing techniques employed by Lloyd to sell his new colorless Hydrastis.

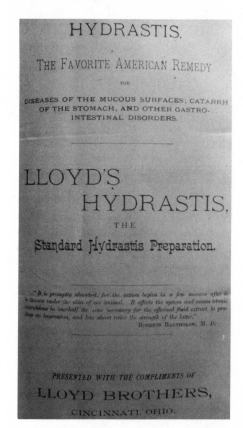

HYDRASTIS.

THE FAVORITE AMERICAN REMEDY

FOR

DISEASES OF THE MUCOUS SURFACES; CATARRH OF THE STOMACH, AND OTHER GASTRO-INTESTINAL DISORDERS.

LLOYD'S HYDRASTIS,

THE

Standard Hydrastis Preparation.

"It is promptly absorbed, for the action begins in a few minutes after it leaves under the skin of an animal. It affects the system and causes tetanic convulsions in one-half the time necessary for the officinal fluid extract to produce an impression, and has about twice the strength of the latter."
ROBERTS BARTHOLOW, M. D.

PRESENTED WITH THE COMPLIMENTS OF

LLOYD BROTHERS,

CINCINNATI, OHIO.

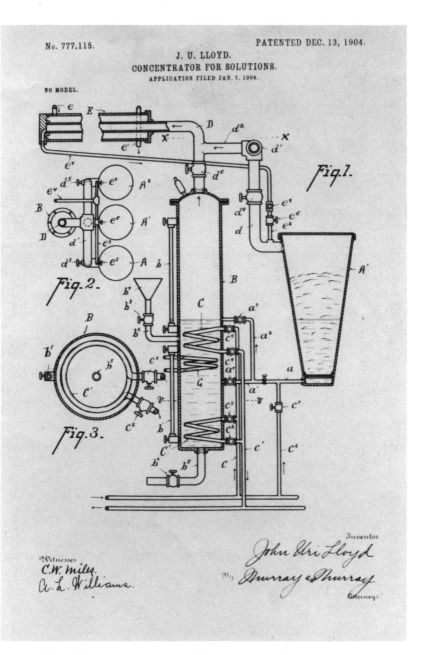

A diagram of Lloyd's famous "cold still" apparatus. The device permitted the extraction of a plant's chemical constituents without the application of heat, which could alter or destroy the therapeutic properties of the material being processed.

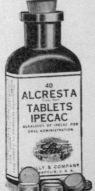
Alcresta advertisement in the *Eclectic Medical Journal* (1916). This buffered ipecac product was one of the practical applications of "Lloyd's reagent." Lloyd sold his process to Eli Lilly, which marketed Alcresta into the 1950s.

THE

CHEMISTRY OF MEDICINES,

PRACTICAL.

A TEXT AND REFERENCE BOOK

FOR THE USE OF

STUDENTS, PHYSICIANS, AND PHARMACISTS,

EMBODYING THE

PRINCIPLES OF CHEMICAL PHILOSOPHY AND THEIR APPLICA-
TION TO THOSE CHEMICALS THAT ARE USED IN MEDICINE
AND IN PHARMACY, INCLUDING ALL THOSE THAT
ARE OFFICINAL IN THE PHARMACOPŒIA OF
THE UNITED STATES.

With Fifty Original Cuts.

By J. U. LLOYD,

Professor of Chemistry in the Eclectic Medical Institute; Professor of
Pharmacy in the Cincinnati College of Pharmacy;
Author of " Elixirs," etc., etc., etc.

EIGHTH EDITION.

———•♦•———

CINCINNATI:
THE ROBERT CLARKE COMPANY,
1897.

Title page of Lloyd's textbook *The Chemistry of Medicines*. An important
contribution to pharmaceutical literature, the book was first published
in 1881 and ran through eight editions.

The original Lloyd Library at 309 West Court Street in Cincinnati. Constructed in 1907–1908, the building served the ever-growing collection for more than fifty years.

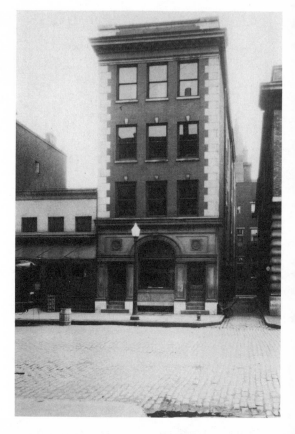

The present Lloyd Library building at 917 Plum Street in Cincinnati. Still on the same corner of Court and Plum, the new building was constructed in 1970 and now faces east.

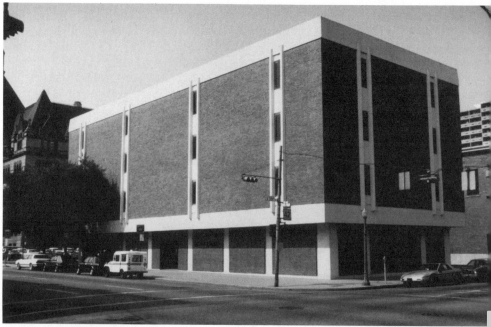

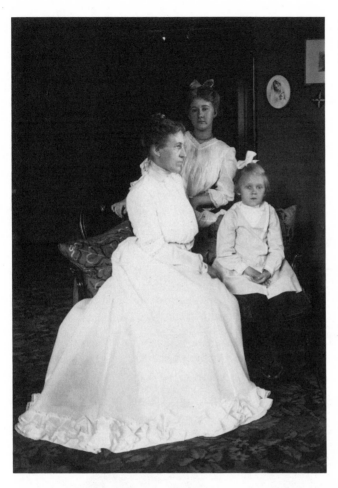

Emma Rouse Lloyd and daughters Anna, *center*, and Dorothy (ca. 1899).

John Uri Lloyd's family (ca. 1890). *Left to right:* Lloyd's mother Sophia, John Uri, son John Thomas, daughter Anna, and wife Emma (known to her close friends as Emmy Lou).

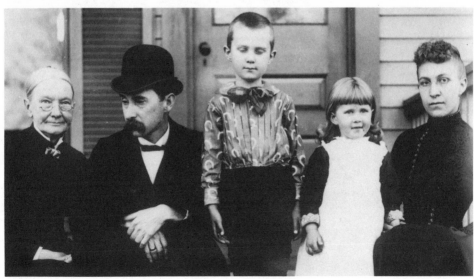

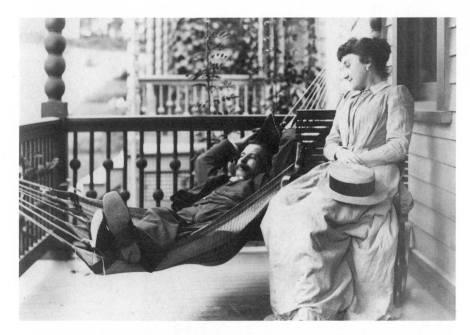

Curtis Lloyd with an unidentified companion. The youngest Lloyd brother was a confirmed bachelor who evidently enjoyed the bachelor's life.

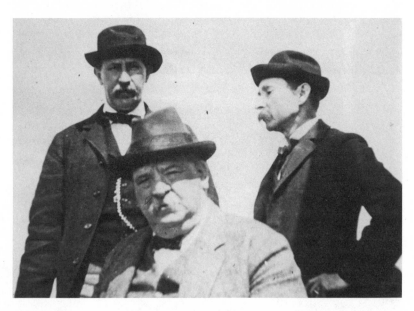

Former president Grover Cleveland, *center*, John Uri Lloyd, *right*, and Cincinnati pharmacist Leroy Brooks on one of their many fishing excursions to Bass Island in Lake Erie.

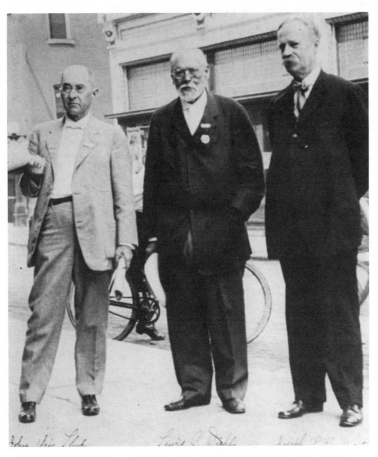

American pharmacy's grand triumvirate, at the APhA annual meeting in Atlantic City (1916). *Left to right:* John Uri Lloyd, C. Lewis Diehl, and Joseph P. Remington.

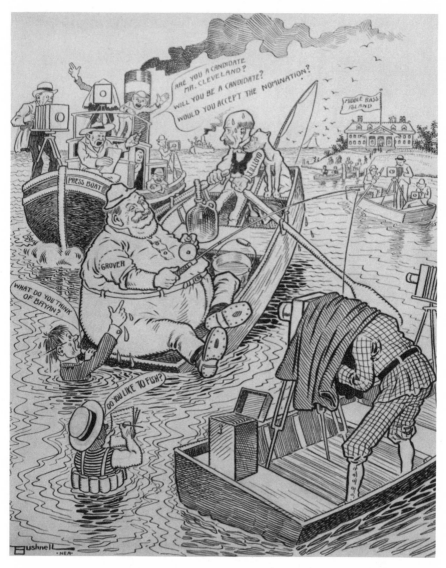

Cartoon depicting a straining "J. U. Lloyd," hounded by the press, rowing his corpulent friend Grover Cleveland toward their favorite fishing spot. Lloyd's political affiliations were well covered by the local newspapers.

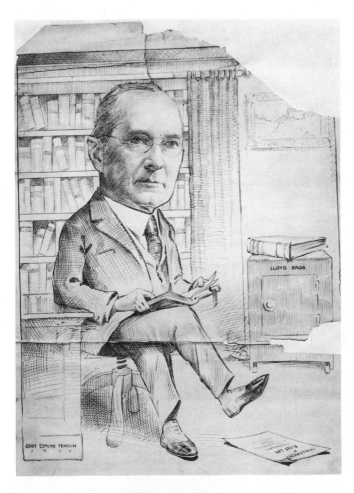

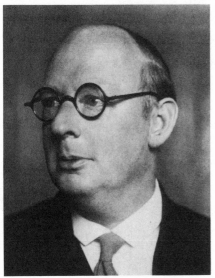

Cartoon depicting Lloyd in his library with the "Indictment of Boss Cox" at his feet. Lloyd's role in the grand jury that indicted George B. Cox in 1911 thrust him into momentary prominence in Cincinnati's politics.

German chemist Wolfgang Ostwald (ca. 1933), who ushered in the new science of modern colloidal chemistry. Ostwald recognized the importance of Lloyd's preliminary work into colloids.

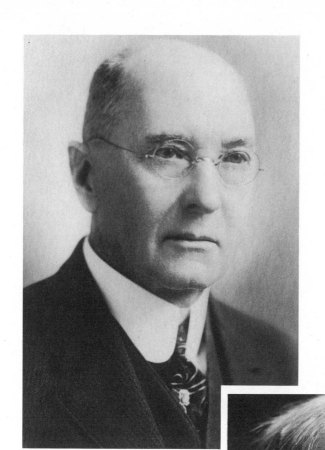

Lloyd in 1920, the year he received American pharmacy's highest honor, the Remington Medal.

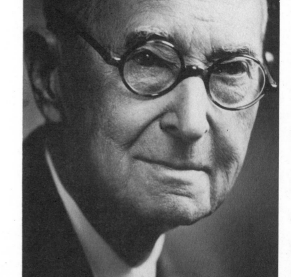

Lloyd in 1935, one year before his death.

5

"The Wizard of American Plant Pharmacy and Chemistry": John Uri Lloyd in His Laboratory

*In an address to the National Eclectic Medical Association at its 1920 meeting in Chicago, James H. Beal (1861–1945), a nationally renowned pharmacist and first recipient of the Remington Medal (1919) for distinguished service to his field, bestowed upon John Uri Lloyd the title of "wizard of American plant pharmacy and chemistry." For Beal, Lloyd was a man who had "enriched with new knowledge every field he has entered, and whose investigations of the colloidal conditions of plant drug constituents have opened up a new world for pharmaceutical exploration."[1]

Beal's praise was not unfounded. Lloyd's laboratory research had long been recognized as yielding important results. "Lloyd was a pioneer in the application of physical chemistry to pharmaceutical techniques," writes John Parascandola in the *Dictionary of Scientific Biography*.[2] The first of these contributions began in 1879 with a series of essays related to the preparation of fluidextracts. These and other published results of Lloyd's lab work made possible important advances in the field of colloidal chemistry. While this constitutes one broad category of Lloyd's scientific accomplishments, the other (really a product of his laboratory research) yielded inventions of apparatus subsequently applied to the pharmaceutical industry. In order to make sense of this latter group, however, it is best to begin with Lloyd's work in applied chemistry.

As chairman of the APhA Committee on Papers and Queries,

Lloyd had the opportunity to consider the major concerns of practicing pharmacists throughout the country. Lloyd was in a particularly advantageous position to do so because of his active research and development with his own Specific Medicines. This gave him a hands-on approach to the practical questions posed to the committee. Query number nineteen initiated what would become a series of articles that offered new approaches to problems in pharmacy and chemistry: "On dissolving solids in water, or in other liquids, a change of bulk is generally produced, consisting in nearly every case in an increase in volume. It is desired to work out a table of the changes of bulk produced by dissolving definite quantities of officinal solids in definite quantities of menstrua [i.e., solvents]."[3]

Lloyd's reply formed an essay titled "On the Conditions Necessary to Successfully Conduct Percolation."[4] Lloyd correctly pointed out that "one of the most frequent operations to be performed by the pharmacist is to separate from the crude materials, offered principally by the vegetable kingdom, active principles from others inert or not desirable." This usually involved maceration (soaking) and percolation (extraction of constituents by descending a solvent over it), both of which were fraught with difficulties in terms of using the appropriate ratios of solids to menstrua.[5] Lloyd's presentation was *not* for the large-scale manufacturer; it was designed so that "every retail pharmacist" had a systematic approach to drugstore percolation. He did this by acknowledging William Procter's earlier use of maceration in conjunction with gravity in a "simple percolation,"[6] but then he went on to demonstrate that the percolation process depended upon a number of factors: The utilization of gravitation, temperature, methods of maceration, types of menstrua, and the type of percolator used all influenced the nature of the finished product. Each of these components was discussed by Lloyd at some length and illustrated in a series of fifteen tables that could be used by every compounding pharmacist as a guide in preparing tinctures and the especially popular fluidextracts.

Yet Lloyd's essay was really only the beginning of what would become extensive excursions into colloidal chemistry. Colloids are simply solid, liquid, or gaseous particles larger than ordinary molecules that are normally dispersed throughout another material. Colloids can be made by mixing a substance (called a dispersed phase) with an appropriate medium (called a dispersing phase). Under the right conditions, water particles mixed in air, for example, form fog (a colloidal suspension); solid pigments mixed in oil or some other liquid base create ink or paint (a sol); and oil, water, and egg yolks produce mayonnaise (a colloidal emulsion). All of these common products (both natural and synthetic) are based upon colloidal principles.[7]

The study of colloids goes back to the late eighteenth century when Tobias Lowitz (1757–1804), a pharmacist-chemist at the Imperial Russian Court Pharmacy, began experimenting with the colorizing and decolorizing properties of charcoal. Lowitz's work earned him the title "father of colloidal chemistry."[8] His early endeavors in this promising new field were continued by others. About 1827, botanist Robert Brown (1773–1858) made important observations concerning the molecular activity of particles that increased when a liquid is heated (dubbed "Brownian movement"). Thomas Graham (1805–1869) performed experiments on the diffusion of gases and the dissolving of salts in solutions that led him, in 1850, to apply two classifications to the kinds of activities he observed of materials in solutions: Those (such as salts) that pass freely through membranes and dissolve quickly in water he called crystalloids; those (such as gelatins and many organic bodies) that form no crystal and diffuse very slowly in solutions he called colloids.[9] Later, William B. Hardy (1864–1934) added to the theory of colloids by showing that when a mildly acid solution was slowly changed to a mildly alkaline solution, the electrical properties of the charged ions become reversed from negative to positive. The so-called isoelectric point at which the charge is completely neutralized causes the solution to become unstable and the colloid to separate and settle, or precipitate, from its solution medium.[10] Today, the importance of this field of applied chemistry extends from synthetics like various fibers and rubber manufacture to biological applications of colloid particle activity to the study of proteins, chromosomes, genes, and even some viruses.

It can readily be seen, then, that Lloyd's work in percolation was bound to impact the colloidal field. The vegetable products being percolated or macerated become the dispersed phase while the menstrua become the dispersing phase. What occurs in terms of the dispersed phases in their menstrua (whether they dissolve or precipitate) is largely a matter of colloidal activity. These questions were extremely important to pharmacists, for they directly affected the quality and shelf life of tinctures and fluidextracts. Thus, Lloyd's activities in this area related more to colloidal solutions than to the suspensions, emulsions, or sols mentioned earlier.

Lloyd got to the heart of the matter in five articles collectively titled "Precipitates in Fluid Extracts."[11] One of the persistent problems with fluidextracts was the fact that they tended over time toward a settling of their constituent parts. Sometimes the precipitated particles could be inert materials that simply affected the cosmetic appearance of the medicine; at other times, however, the precipitates could be the active ingredients affecting the therapeutic value of the remedy itself. In either case, the product would often become so altered that no amount of shaking of the bottle would return the solution to its original state, and it would have to be discarded. It is in this context that Lloyd opened his first paper on precipitates in pharmaceutical preparations: "Still prone to change upon standing, one of the results is the production of precipitates, and to a very great extent these precipitates result from the reaction between menstruum and powder during the act of percolation, to the consideration of which this article is devoted. Before, however, entering into the line of argument I shall assume that, as a class, precipitates are objectionable, whether composed of inert materials or of active medicinal agents."[12]

Lloyd noted and discussed at some length five different factors affecting precipitation: oxidation, change of solvent strength with evaporation of the menstruum, change in temperature, chemical change, and light. The paper did not resolve the problem of precipitation with a simple formula for its elimination. It did, however, offer considerable details on the reactions that would take place under various stages of the percolation process, *and* it offered some suggestions on eliminating precipitation of the most important agents in the solution as a whole. After outlining and describing a series of eleven experiments that he had conducted related to precipitation, Lloyd concluded, "I must say that it does not seem probable that we shall ever, by percolation alone, succeed in making a line of permanent fluid extracts from dry plants. The most important step, then, is to adapt our menstruum so that it may hold in solution the *medicinal* principles of each plant, and thus render the precipitate which forms inert; for the precipitate *will* follow."[13]

Lloyd continued his study of precipitates in a paper read at the fourth session of the 1882 annual APhA meeting in Niagara Falls, New York. Pointing out that precipitation was a more or less continuous process due both to physical manipulations of solutions through percolation and to natural causes such as gravity, Lloyd demonstrated that precipitates could never be totally eliminated from fluidextracts or tinctures and that in time some precipitation would occur in virtually all of these solutions. The response of leading APhA members was overwhelmingly favorable. Joseph P. Remington cited the importance of studying percolation and expressed his appreciation to Lloyd, as did others in attendance who saw in this paper the complex nature of the percolation process. Lloyd won his first Ebert Prize for original research in pharmacy for this essay.

The last three articles read at the annual APhA meetings for 1883 through 1885 considered other types of precipitates, such as those that exhibit crystalline formations on the surface or above certain fluid preparations like sodium chloride and tinctures of bittersweet *(Solanum dulcamara)* and sea wrack *(Fucus vesiculosus)*, and the influence of capillarity in separating a solvent from dissolved matter. While Lloyd's investigations in these areas did not solve the problem of precipitation per se, they did offer some new approaches to the handling of fluid preparations. Perhaps the three most important of these were summarized in his 1884 essay as three postulates:

1st. Liquids can be separated from solids held in solution, without evaporating the liquid or precipitating the solid in an insoluble condition.

2nd. Liquids can be separated from each other.

3rd. Chemical combinations even can be broken without calling upon such recognized dissociating powers as high or low temperature, or the action of reagents.[14]

Lloyd's separation principles and ongoing interest in processing solutions allowed him to build upon this work and develop new methods for assaying alkaloids like aconite *(Aconitum* spp.), belladonna *(Atropa belladonna)*, coca *(Erythroxylum coca)*, guanara *(Paullinia cupana)*, and lobelia *(Lobelia inflata)*. In a series of essays published in 1891, Lloyd would again earn an Ebert Prize for his "schemes of assaying."[15] The big discovery lay ahead, however.

Not until he accidentally stumbled upon a unique application of fuller's earth some nineteen years later would it become apparent that these earlier studies could yield a truly new and special use. In a paper that earned him his third Ebert Prize for distinguished research in the field, Lloyd described this process of discovery in detail:

> In the winter of 1910, calling to my experimental laboratory Mr. William J. Miller, foreman of the technical laboratory [of Lloyd Brothers] that takes my special care, I said: "Make a mixture of five parts berberine sulphate, with ninety-five parts fullers' earth. Bring it to a putty like condition with water, working it well in a Wedgwood mortar to a complete and thorough admixture, then dry the product, powder it, and bring me a sample."
>
> Within a reasonable time, a powder having the bright yellow color of berberine was brought to my desk. It was practically odorless, and seemed to be an intimately incorporated mixture of the two substances. Placing some of it upon my tongue, I found it tasteless! Sending for Mr. Miller I asked:
>
> Are you sure that this mixture is as I directed, sulphate of berberine and fullers' earth only?
>
> "Exactly as directed," he replied.
>
> Taking a small amount of the mixture, I digested it with diluted sulphuric acid, and filtered it. The filtrate was colorless, and gave no alkaloidal reaction. The residue on the filter paper retained its full berberine yellow color, but was tasteless.
>
> "Send for a sample of the fullers' earth used." It also came, and then I took the subject in hand.
>
> I made a mixture of berberine sulphate and fullers' earth, in the proportions aforenamed, added the same to distilled water, agitated the mixture well, and filtered. Behold! the filtrate passed colorless and devoid of alkaloid. I placed some of the residue upon the filter paper, on my tongue. It was tasteless. This mixture likewise, when digested with diluted acid, and filtered, gave no evidence of an alkaloid being present.

Next I took, successively, other alkaloidal salts, such as those of morphine, quinine, cocaine, etc., submitted them to the same manipulation, and found that *all alkaloids experimented with* produced insoluble compounds, and that all (brucine excepted) were practically tasteless. I also discovered that the reaction was nearly instantaneous.[16]

This discovery was of considerable importance. Alkaloids have had a long history of medicinal uses. Although they form a class of highly toxic vegetable products (the tropane alkaloids, for example, form some of the so-called classic poisons employed in ancient, legendary assassination attempts and incorporated into Shakespeare's plays),[17] they also represent some of the first active agents scientifically extracted from plants for medicinal use. Strychnine, first isolated in 1818, was used as a heart and respiratory stimulant; in 1820 quinine produced from *Cinchona calisaya* was used for treating malaria; and in 1831 the systematic extraction of atropine from *Atropa belladona* led to its use as an antispasmodic and heart stimulant.[18]

Lloyd's discovery that berberine (an especially bitter-tasting yellow constituent of barberry) could be made tasteless and colorless was the first report of a buffered alkaloid: the fuller's earth had neutralized the base without appreciably altering the alkalinity of the solution. For this reason, Lloyd had not found (as he had first thought) a reliable antidote for all types of alkaloidal poisoning. Nevertheless, Martin I. Wilbert and Professor A. B. Stevens felt that such a discovery held some therapeutic promise. In particular, Wilbert correctly concluded that with the application of this process to a product like nux vomica (from a tree, *Strychnos nux-vomica*, native to Southeast Asia yielding strychnine), the action of strychnine could be held in abeyance until reaching the "alkaline secretions of the bowels." Patients could in theory avoid the horrible bitter taste and even the occasional stomach upset associated with the ingestion of certain otherwise toxic products if they were simply buffered in this manner. Dr. Sigmund Waldbott, a chemist who was a close friend and associate of Lloyd, found that the active constituent in the fuller's earth that caused this buffering action was hydrous aluminum silicate, a naturally occurring group of substances containing various amounts of aluminum and silicon oxides, dubbed simply Lloyd's reagent because of his discovery. Lloyd's work in the areas of preparing fluidextracts and colloid chemistry had come together to produce a new and useful process. "In making and extracting this compound from the forms of clay that I have investigated," he told APhA members in 1914, "I have found it desirable, as nearly as possible, to bring the abstracted and hydrated material into a colloidal condition, in which form, it has an intense affinity for alkaloids and alkaloidal salts."[19] H. M. Gordon and Jay Kaplin compared this fuller's earth reagent with charcoal (a substance commonly used in the adsorption of alkaloids) and found that "while in the scope of adsorbable substances charcoal probably excels Lloyd's reagent, in velocity of adsorption of alkaloids, the reagent far surpasses charcoal.[20] The complete removal of alkaloids by means of charcoal usually requires digestion with continuous shaking for several hours, while adsorption by Lloyd's reagent," they concluded, "is complete within a few minutes."[21] Not surprisingly, Lloyd's reagent found its way into the pharmaceutical industry in 1913. A press release to eclectic physicians signed by Lloyd on November 17 read, in part, as follows:

> Arrangements have this day been consummated whereby the firm of Eli Lilly & Company, Indianapolis, Indiana, have acquired the sole privilege of making and marketing the alkaloidal precipitant known as "LLOYD'S REAGENT," which is a form of hydrous aluminum silicate. They have also acquired the right to manufacture all commercial products, medicinal or otherwise, in tablets, triturates, pills, capsules, and pharmaceutical preparations generally. Whoever may be concerned in this subject, or in acquiring privileges and rights under the patents granted the undersigned, whether at home or abroad, is hereby referred to the aforenamed firm, Eli Lilly & Company, the undersigned being relieved from all commercial connection with the subject. . . .
>
> It should be stated that inasmuch as the reagent has become commonly known as "LLOYD'S REAGENT," that term, in connection with the scientific name "HYDROUS ALUMINUM SILICATE," will hereafter be accepted as the name of the reagent itself, which will be so labeled, the short term "ALCRESTA" being a trade mark term, its application being lim-

In 1915 Dr. Bernard Fantus, a professor of pharmacology and therapeutics at the University of Illinois, verified many of the early claims for the reagent.[23] Taking notice of Lloyd's previous work, Fantus subjected fuller's earth to intensive analysis and determined that because of the reagent's adsorptive properties the substance "has antidotal value in morphin, cocain, nicotin, and ipecac poisoning." Lloyd's bitter disappointment that he had *not* found a universal antidote for alkaloid poisoning (merely a buffering agent) was at least partly alleviated by Fantus's confirmation that the addition of tartaric acid increased the antidotal value of his reagent. Fantus concluded that while the power of adsorption varied in different fuller's earths, "Lloyd's reagent possesses this power to the highest degree."

By 1916 Eli Lilly was actively promoting "Alcresta Tablets of Ipecac" for amoebic dysentery and pyorrhea. Lilly described its product as tablets that "disintegrate readily in the stomach, but do not release the alkaloids until the alkaline intestinal secretions are reached," thus causing "no gastric disturbance."[24] The theory behind this medication was that the ipecac would work against the amoebic infection while the buffering action of the hydrous aluminum silicate protected the stomach and generally ameliorated the harsh effects of the toxin. Prescribed by eclectic *and* regular physicians, Alcresta had a comparatively long career in the pharmaceutical industry; the Eli Lilly company continued to manufacture Alcresta Tablets of Ipecac through 1956.[25]

A summary of events leading up to the development of Lloyd's reagent shows the sometimes curious and often twisted processes of discovery: In a series of experiments originally designed to eliminate precipitates in fluidextracts and tinctures, Lloyd made new contributions to colloidal chemistry and in so doing discovered a reagent that effectively caused a precipitate action when fuller's earth was brought to a colloidal condition.

Lloyd's contribution did not go unnoticed by others. Atherton Seidell utilized the adsorption properties of fuller's earth in extracting B-complex vitamins from yeast, a process he patented in February of 1916.[26] Wolfgang Ostwald (1883–1943), a lecturer at the University of

Leipzig who gained recognition for colloidal chemistry as an independent field and who led the discipline as the editor of the influential *Kolloidchemische Beihefte*, was so impressed with Lloyd's work that he translated and reprinted his articles on precipitates in his journal.[27] Ostwald praised the essays in his introduction as researches containing "truly exemplary insight" into pharmaceutical and chemical phenomena not replicated "even in the handbooks and pharmacopoeia." (See appendix 3 for the complete introduction.) In Ostwald's opinion, there was not "anything which even approximates the complete, detailed, copious discussion . . . than is to be found in the present treatise of J. U. Lloyd."[28]

An acknowledgment of this caliber bestowed upon an American pharmacist by a ranking member of the German scientific community was no small matter. During this period, Germany and indeed much of western Europe was on the cutting edge of scientific research and development on virtually every front. Ostwald's acclamation of Lloyd's work was also reiterated in his book-length treatise on colloidal chemistry.[29] Historian George Urdang has rightly called this "one of the greatest tributes paid to an American scientist by European science."[30]

Ostwald was not the first European scientist to be aware of Lloyd's rising stature in the American pharmaceutical community. The famous Swiss pharmacist Burkhard Reber (1848–1926) included Lloyd in his *Gallery of Prominent Therapists and Pharmacognosists of the Present* more than a decade earlier in 1894.[31] Reber referred to Lloyd as "a sharp observer and careful experimenter," with the quality of his work "distinguished particularly through the reliability of the results." Noting Lloyd's prolific pen and his pragmatic approach to the discipline, Reber suggested that a collection of Lloyd's publications would "offer an important gold mine of information for the practical apothecary, historian of pharmacy, and the producers and wholesalers."

Despite Reber's high praise, it was not he who made Ostwald aware of Lloyd's work with colloids. The interesting means by which the German chemist was alerted to Lloyd's essays touching on colloidal activity sheds light on the personality of their author. One would have suspected that Ostwald discovered Lloyd's work on his own through the pages of the *Proceedings of the American Pharmaceutical Association*. As a young student, Ostwald spent three years as a research assistant to Jacques Loeb

(1859–1924), the noted researcher in animal tropisms, parthenogenesis, and colloidal activity in proteins at the University of California at Berkeley.[32] In this active academic environment, Ostwald would have had access to a wide range of scientific literature. Despite this fact, a publication only marginally related to Ostwald and Loeb's research interests could easily have escaped their notice.

Yet it was clearly Lloyd who pointed out his previous work to the chemist. These essays were shown to Ostwald when he visited Lloyd's library in April of 1914. But simply showing the essays to Ostwald was not enough; Lloyd assembled all of his essays together under the title *A Study in Pharmacy* and added a revealing introduction stating that this was "made for Dr. Ostwald by the author." "A few copies, (twelve only), of this print, are issued in advance," Lloyd added, "for the purpose of placing the old time data in the hands of Dr. Ostwald. The author begs you to accept this, (one of the advance copies), with his compliments, as a token of his regard."[33] It was probably from this dedicatory reprinting that Ostwald selected Lloyd's material for the *Kolloidchemische Beihefte*. Such obvious self-promotion should not suggest that his work on precipitates and colloids was unworthy of republication to the European scholarly community in an important scientific journal but that Lloyd was unquestionably persistent—even opportunistic—in publicizing his work.

Lloyd's reputation in the laboratory does not rest upon his work in colloidal chemistry alone. His activities, it must be remembered, all stemmed from the desire to perfect manufacturing processes at his own plant. For this reason, Lloyd's studies led him to develop improved apparatus for extraction of vegetable products. One of the most important involved the invention of a "concentrator for solutions" that subsequently became known as Lloyd's "cold still" extractor.

Lloyd's cold still emerged out of concerns that heat during the percolation process caused a dissociation of a plant's active constituents, thus lessening, and in some cases destroying, the potency and efficacy of the desired agent or agents. This problem was well known and discussed in the first edition of *Remington's Practice of Pharmacy*.[34] Lloyd too had long been concerned with the effects of temperature in processing medicinal plant products and had devoted considerable attention to this issue.[35] His solution was embodied in patent number 777,115 lodged with the U.S.

patent office on December 13, 1904. Lloyd described his concentrator as follows: "The object of my invention is an apparatus for making solutions, such as extracts and abstracts, whereby the substance held in solution is not changed by heat, by which the strength of the solution may be changed readily to suit the case, in which the alcohol or other menstruum remaining in the waste may be recovered readily for use again."[36]

By 1909 Lloyd's concentrator was in use in England. F. B. Kilmer demonstrated the practical implications of this pharmaceutical innovation by describing the superior benefits of the machine at the laboratories of Johnson and Johnson to Frederick B. Power at London's Burroughs, Wellcome:

> In brief I may state that I consider the apparatus and method the most perfect that I have ever seen, and in making this statement I would say that I have had occasion to be familiar with the methods used in the larger laboratories of the United States, and some of those used abroad.
>
> One of the particular features of the apparatus is the space occupied. In our former method we used percolators holding about 250 pounds each; as an accompaniment we had large tanks for mixing menstruum, moistening the drug and work of like character, which filled a room 33 × 72 feet, and some tanks occupying other stories in the building. Beginning two years ago we installed the Lloyd apparatus which we have since enlarged to a size of about double our former capacity, and the whole apparatus and work is concentrated in a room less than 30 feet square. . . .
>
> Further than this there is the remarkable saving in alcohol. Under our old method we had apparatus in the way of tanks and automatic feeding appliances to carry alcohol to the percolators, etc., but under the best conditions the waste of alcohol was very large. At the present time our loss of alcohol is so small that we do not take it into account in reckoning the cost of our product.
>
> We manufacture with this apparatus only the solid extract of belladonna. The capacity of our apparatus is six thousand

pounds of the drug. We produce about 350 pounds of solid extract per week, and could produce much more if necessary.

I have been quite interested and surprised at the increased yield of alkaloid. Formerly we only obtained about 80% of the theoretical amount of alkaloid of belladonna, this for the reason that we found the continued extraction involved such an expenditure of labor as to be unprofitable. Under our present method we obtain, as our records show, fully 100% of alkaloid. . . .

In other words, the extract seems to be practically unchanged and fully represents the drug. I was impressed with this fact in examining some extracts made from aromatic plants in the Lloyd Laboratory.[37]

With such obvious advantages, Lloyd's cold still quickly became widely adopted in large-scale manufacturing. By 1926 an extensive entry on Lloyd's extractor with detailed instructions for its use appeared in *Remington's Practice of Pharmacy*, a testimony to its general acceptance and use in the pharmaceutical industry. For almost fifty years, some discussion of the Lloyd extractor was carried in the pages of *Remington's*. Nevertheless, by 1948 certain disadvantages to its use caused a slow waning of interest in the apparatus: "The Lloyd extractor cannot be employed where mixed solvents are used,"[38] it was noted. Reiterating this limitation, the last mention of the Lloyd extractor appeared in the 1975 edition of *Remington's*.[39] Besides this, the general trend of pharmaceuticals away from natural products toward synthetics made Lloyd's extractor a thing of the past. Still, it was a long and distinguished career for one machine in an extremely dynamic industry.

Along with Lloyd's extractor, a number of other products were spawned from Lloyd's lab. Archival records indicate no less than sixteen U.S. patents for a variety of percolators, concentrators, purifiers, and condensers for the processing of solutions and alkaloidal salts, plus an assortment of medical appliances.[40] Many of these represented improvements and modifications to his original cold still patent of 1904, but some were unrelated and even preceded his most famous invention. His "Vial or Medicine Bottle," for example, was deposited with the patent office in 1899 and was designed to deliver its contents in measured drops. In 1915

Lloyd developed an atropine sulfate preparation from jimson weed *(Datura stramonium)*. Eli Lilly manufactured stropine from this plant using Lloyd's reagent and had exclusive rights to provide this product to the U.S. government for the treatment of eye wounds during World War I. Another significant product of Lloyd's lab was his patented "Medicine Dropper or Syringe" developed in 1928, a natural adjunct to his vial in that its design allowed for a more precise and efficient dosage delivery of ophthalmic medication.

Amid this dazzling array of test tubes, Bunsen burners, beakers, retorts, and the attendant concoctions emanating from a conglomeration of concentrators, purifiers, and percolators, the wizard of American plant chemistry and pharmacy was in his true element. Here, surrounded by a bouquet of pungent aromas emanating from the volatile oils of vegetable products ever in process, Lloyd could focus on a wide range of practical problems facing his colleagues and apply a pragmatic, hands-on approach to solving them. Within this environment of experimentation and investigation, Lloyd established himself as a pharmaceutical innovator of major proportions. In the laboratory, Lloyd clearly surpassed *all* his eclectic comrades, past and present.

Beal's reference to Lloyd as a "wizard" suggests the compelling association with the more famous "Wizard of Menlo Park." In his laboratory, Lloyd does indeed emerge as a kindred spirit to Thomas Alva Edison (1847–1931). Although there is no evidence that they knew one another, they were contemporaries. More important, both approached problems in much the same way: Tireless workers, Lloyd and Edison could become obsessed with difficult questions and would often labor long and hard until a project was successfully concluded. Distinctively American, their work was characterized more by ingenuity than by scholarly analysis; Lloyd and Edison solved their problems by producing physical manifestations of their resolution. Edison's fascination with new communications media, for example, produced the kinetograph and phonograph, and the difficulty of finding a durable filament that could emit light without extinguishing was ultimately resolved with the incandescent light bulb. Likewise, out of Lloyd's determination to develop purer fluidextracts and tinctures came his discoveries of colloidal principles that led to a new reagent used in creating Alcresta; and from the problems associated with heat in the processing of medicinal plants came the cold still extractor. Francis Jehl, Edison's lab assistant and companion of fifty years, once remarked that the Menlo Park laboratory was an arcade of inventions in progress where "sentiments were magnified almost to the verge of hallucination, lighted up with a bewitching glimmer—like an alchemist's den."[41] This could just as easily have been said of Lloyd's lab in Cincinnati.

Yet despite their pragmatism, both men were bibliophiles. Edison kept a standing account at Brentano's bookstore in Manhattan.[42] But where Edison ordered hundreds of dollars of books per month (a large sum in those days), Lloyd ordered thousands of dollars of books per month (an astronomical sum in those days). Their reading habits differed too. Where Edison read a diffuse assortment of books feeding "his indiscriminately hungry mind,"[43] Lloyd read books, both new and old, almost exclusively related to pharmacy and botany. Lloyd's leisure reading included ancient treatises on alchemy, long-forgotten pharmacopeias and dispensatories, and classic medical works by Dioscorides and Apuleius Barbarus. For Lloyd, a library was like a toolbox to be filled with materials that might prove useful in completing some task related to his profession. This sharp focus and disciplined collection development would yield his greatest achievement of all: his amassing a specialized collection of research materials on phytomedicine and pharmacy. In fact, almost from the day that he began with H. M. Merrell in 1871, Lloyd engaged in one continuous activity: The wizard was building his library.

6

Building a Workshop: John Uri Lloyd and His Library

Justin Winsor (1831–1897), the Harvard librarian who led his profession as the first president of the American Library Association, proclaimed that "a great library should be a workshop as well as a repository. It should teach the methods of thorough research, and cultivate in readers the habit of seeking the original sources of learning."[1] Indeed, as Kenneth Brough has pointed out, the metaphor of the library as the scholar's "workshop" and "laboratory" was a popular and persistent one at the turn of the century. Few repositories in the world have from their very inception epitomized this conception of the library more than the collection amassed by John Uri Lloyd during the last quarter of the nineteenth century.

Lloyd indicated in very clear terms that his was a *working* library: "an outgrowth of the necessity for information concerning the American Materia Medica and the Eclectic preparations, which had become a special study of its founders."[2] Later librarians have been fond of pointing out that three books formed the embryo of what would evolve into today's two-hundred-thousand-volume library of international renown: George Fownes's *Chemistry*; Parrish's *Introduction to Practical Pharmacy*; and a small, vest-pocket Bible. These books comprised young John's library as an apprentice under William J. M. Gordon.[3] Yet Lloyd himself pointed to his connection with John King and eclecticism as the beginning of a systematic amassing of a specialized collection in pharmacy. When Lloyd agreed to take charge of H. M. Merrell's laboratory and devote himself exclusively to investigating plants for their medicinal potentials, the acquisition of supporting research materials became of paramount importance. Recounting in third person the procedures initiated to secure works in this field, Lloyd told members of the historical section of the APhA that "It was found that the literature in this direction was very much scattered, and in order to acquaint himself with the record of the past, it was essential that he should obtain for reference a complete file of the standard Eclectic publication known as the *Eclectic Medical Recorder*, together with its antecedent (seven volumes, 1836 to 1848) of the *Western Medical Reformer*."[4] The systematic search that followed yielded much more than these two series. By means of advertisements placed in the professional literature, along with the help of John Milton Scudder and John King, John and Ashley Lloyd collected books and journals from all over the country. This formed the core of the Lloyd Library collection. "Thus it was that, without any thought of doing more than fortifying their own work and investigations in what was then largely an untrodden field, they together laid the foundations for this special library."

The development of the library would take a decided turn toward botany when Curtis Gates Lloyd joined the Lloyd Brothers operations in 1886. Curtis had by then developed a passion for plant taxonomy, but his short stint at the Standard Publishing Company in Cincinnati had also awakened the bibliophile in him. Curtis took it upon himself to broaden his original charge as an active partner with the Lloyd Brothers firm to include not only the field investigation of medicinal plants but also the acquisition of books on this subject, plus botany and his personal favorite, mycology.

It was an excellent partnership; the library grew rapidly with John as ex officio director and Curtis as the traveling collection-development agent. Close to home, John began assembling the infrastructure for a growing library. He designated Sigmund Waldbott (1865–1950), a German-born graduate of the University of Bern who had been the assistant chemist at Lloyd Brothers since 1893, to function as the part-time librarian for the burgeoning collection. It was about this time that, just prior to his death, John King donated his sizable library to John Lloyd. Meanwhile, Curtis began searching the world for valuable books to add to the collection, an activity that coincided with frequent to trips to Kew Gardens and other leading botanical centers throughout Europe.

Here, Curtis effectively combined his training as a pharmacist, his interest in botany, and his love of books to become an outstanding buyer for the Lloyd collection.

As the shelves continued to swell at the Lloyd Brothers manufacturing plant, it became clear that a separate facility would be needed to house the collection. In 1901 a building at 224 West Court Street in Cincinnati was purchased for this purpose, and John's accumulation of three thousand books on pharmacy, chemistry, and vegetable materia medica were combined with Curtis's books on botany.[5] But the structure was inadequate from the beginning, and by 1902 John was announcing the completion of a new building: "The past year found the Library filled to overflowing with books, and in order to meet the urgent demands of the work, the old building was torn down and a new, four-story structure, the full size of the lot took its place. . . . With renewed energies do we now expect to devote ourselves to this library work, not neglecting our business, of course, and such duties as connected therewith."[6]

The library was gaining more than just new quarters, however. In 1901 Waldbott left his post as librarian to assume the head of the chemistry department at the Ohio Mechanic's Institute. Unfortunately, Waldbott had not executed his duties at the library particularly well; the library's need for bibliographic control and collection management had not been well served by the German's scholarly interests. Writing privately to his friend and colleague at the University of Wisconsin, Edward Kremers, Lloyd admitted in retrospect the error of turning his library over to the care of a chemist:

> I wish confidentially to say to you that the mistake of our
> life as concerns the library was that of making a librarian of a
> man interested in the contents of the library. He should be interested only in the compilation of those books not in their field
> of action. Take for example, Dr. Waldbott, talented even beyond
> compare, when he would take a book, instead of studying the
> title page and making his notes concerning its place in the library and then laying it down, he would become involved in
> the contents of the book, and read and read and read detail[ed]
> subjects that were in it, putting in sometimes a whole day on a

single volume. This to you in confidence. My failure to comprehend that fact has been to great disadvantage as concerned
our library, which is now, however, rapidly taking on a systematic form and will when completed be all that we had hoped it
would be.[7]

The promise of the new facilities was matched by the enthusiasm
of the newly installed librarian, William Holden (1839–1913). This former captain and Civil War veteran of the Eighteenth Ohio Infantry had
been the librarian at Marietta College, a small liberal arts school situated
along the Ohio River. By March of 1903, Lloyd was praising Holden's
work. In the same letter to Edward Kremers in which he decried the
deficiencies of Waldbott, Lloyd told the Wisconsin professor that, under
the captain's direction, the library "is being systematically and perfectly
arranged." In fact, he added, "Should you visit it now, you would be
struck at once with the difference between the plant that you saw when
you were here and the present." In an effort to make the ever-growing
collection accessible, Holden persevered for several years; Lloyd told Kremers that the captain and a few assistants "have been for over two years
constantly working on this catalogue."[8] The classification scheme was
unique. Essentially an alphabetic scheme, the system comprised from one
to three characters in combination, interfiled by a simple alphanumeric
system commonly used in libraries that was devised by Charles Ammi
Cutter of the Boston Athenaeum. Black letter combinations were used
for botany, horticulture, and related fields, and red letters for medicine,
pharmacy, and chemistry.[9] While Holden and his assistant Edith Wycoff
were well intentioned, the creation of a special classification arrangement was rather unfortunate. Despite all their efforts, the scheme itself
was not especially flexible, and eventually the carefully devised divisions
and subdivisions could not keep pace with the rapid growth of speciali-
zation in any of the areas it was designed to classify. So long as the collection did not become too large (in excess of seventy-five thousand
volumes or so) this did not pose a major problem. In time, however, the
awkward features of a purely alphabetic system made themselves apparent, with numerous titles receiving the same classification and Cutter
assignments.

This classification problem is all the more unfortunate because such work was unnecessary and counterproductive. Melvil Dewey (1851–1931) had published his decimal system in 1876 under the title *A Classification and Subject Index for Cataloguing and Arranging the Books and Pamphlets of a Library*. This was just the first in his many innovations helping to usher in a modern era of professionalized library management.[10] As early as 1880, Dr. John Shaw Billings (1838–1913) had set the standard in medical library organization by transforming a mishmash of some 1,600 volumes under the army surgeon general's office in 1865 into a well-categorized and carefully indexed collection of 50,000 books and 60,000 pamphlets comprising the Army Medical Library, the core of which would eventually become the National Library of Medicine in 1956.[11] There were also changes transpiring at the Library of Congress under the energetic newly installed librarian Herbert Putnam (1861–1955). When Putnam announced to four hundred libraries and seventeen state library commissions the first nationwide shared cataloging system with the distribution of printed LC cards on October 26, 1901, Holden should have taken notice.[12] Had the Lloyd Library adopted a more widely accepted classification scheme from the beginning, a considerable amount of reclassification could have been avoided in the future. As it was, Holden's system was idiosyncratic and kept the library out of the mainstream of modern bibliographic control methods being ushered in by leading librarians like Dewey, Billings, and Putnam.

Such was definitely *not* the case with its collection development techniques, however. Armed with detailed "want lists" compiled by Holden, Curtis (himself a knowledgeable pharmacist turned botanist) combed the antiquarian bookshops of Europe in search of appropriate titles for the library. This sharp and exceptionally informed focus on pharmacy and botany (and especially phytomedicine) helped the library to acquire the historically significant and important books in these fields. Despite Holden's questionable classification skills, what his comprehensive catalog index lacked as a finding aid and bibliographic control tool it more than made up for in acquisitions. Caswell Mayo explains this remarkably efficient system in detail:

> The catalogue prepared by Captain Holden was not only a
> catalogue of books found in the library, but embraced all titles
> that could be gathered from available sources that came within

the scope of the subjects covered by the library. From this catalogue, Curtis, when traveling, was furnished with various "purchasing lists," such as a French list, comprising all French titles
named in the catalogue with marks indicating those already
possessed by the library, a similar German list, etc. While traveling in Europe, Curtis visited the great book centers, Paris,
Berlin, Leipzig, London, Stockholm, etc., and by means of these
lists, which were checked over by the dealers, was enabled to
buy books in quantity, with little personal trouble of detail
work. As books were purchased they were marked temporarily
on the purchasing lists. When the lists were returned to the library in Cincinnati, and the books were received, a permanent
record was made on both catalogue and purchasing list. This
plan was evolved by Captain Holden, whose systematic work
can not be too highly praised.

It was customary for the Librarian to purchase such new
American books as came within the library's scope [often at the
suggestion of John Lloyd], also to buy as opportunity offered
of the older American publications as were not already on the
shelves, the purchase of all foreign books being left to Curtis
during his travels abroad. This was necessary to prevent dupli-
cation.[13]

The books were purchased with the proceeds of Lloyd's novels,
Stringtown on the Pike in particular. This local color tale was immensely
popular and netted Lloyd a tidy sum. At its first release late in 1900, the
local newspapers announced that 10,000 copies of the book were sold
before it was even printed.[14] By February of 1901, there were 50,000 in
print, selling for $1.50 each, with additional printings in England by
Holder and Stoughton. While it might have been unsubstantiated hype,
one newspaper claimed, "The royalty offered by the concern [Dodd,
Mead] to Mr. Lloyd is higher than any ever paid Mark Twain or any
American author."[15] Although the article does not give a figure, a conservative estimate would be that Lloyd received at least $6,000 in
American sales alone for *Stringtown*.[16] This may not sound like a huge
sum in terms of a straight dollar amount, but such a figure represented
roughly six times the annual income of a skilled worker during the

period.[17] The bottom line is: *Stringtown* bought a lot of books for the library. By early 1902, Lloyd could publicly announce that "it gives me pleasure to inform you that the returns from my outside literary ventures, which were largely the result of recreative hours, a kind of rest diversion, have given us an unexpected fund, by which to increase the book department."[18]

And increase it did. The period from 1902 to 1909 saw the shelves of the Lloyd Library fill with rare books from Europe. Scarce pharmacopeias and dispensatories, rare herbals, and much sought after taxonomic treatises on botany began to pour into the library. As Curtis scoured the overseas bookshops, John Uri wrote to Edward Kremers of his purchases. In September of 1905, for example, Lloyd told Kremers that "a consignment of books is now in our Custom House, some 1,200 volumes, from Germany,"[19] and again, less than a month later, Lloyd mentioned the addition of another 2,500 volumes from his brother in Europe.[20] By 1909 both the facilities and the collection had grown rapidly. John proudly told Kremers, "I wish you could visit the library in its new home. You would scarcely recognize its new surroundings, and in the large increase in books that has been made since you were here. Several other large purchases are now on their way from Europe, where my brother, C. G. Lloyd, is constantly picking up whatever he finds in the way of completing various departments of the Library."[21]

The construction of a "new home" was almost a foregone conclusion from the completion of the 1902 building. Despite the fact that John had suggested to Curtis that two floors be added for expansion, his brother had insisted that the original plans were sufficient. Nevertheless, John was complaining by July of 1903 that on the second and fourth stories "the only place left now for books is the floor" and that with purchases by the coming fall "the entire space of the Lloyd Library will be filled, necessitating us to arrange immediately for additional room."[22] This was accomplished by retaining the 1902 structure and converting it into an herbarium and repository for the mycological and botanical works that Curtis deemed appropriate while an entirely new four-story building was constructed in 1907–1908 at 309 West Court Street. Now there was housing exclusively for books, and pains were taken to assure room for expansion. This building was approximately 22 by 72 feet, with room for 6,253 linear feet of shelving. At full capacity, the Lloyd

Library at 309 West Court Street could hold an estimated 98,000 volumes in 11,413 linear feet of shelving. This would remain the permanent location of the library for more than sixty years until it too became insufficient to hold the expanding collection.

This was not actually Lloyd's original plan. Extant correspondence clearly indicates at least an ostensible desire to relocate the library as part of a larger academic institution at some point. Undoubtedly in response to Lloyd's search for another location for his library, a flurry of letters arrived in 1904 from schools seeking the collection. The provost of the University of Pennsylvania, for example, touted the benefits the library in Philadelphia, long a center of medical and pharmaceutical activity;[23] Oscar Oldberg of the College of Pharmacy at Northwestern University told Lloyd that "no other institution would take greater pride in maintaining it and increasing it in perpetuity;"[24] Burris Jenkins, president of Kentucky University, pled his case for locating the library in the Bluegrass;[25] Professor Coville, a botanist, suggested that the Lloyd Library become affiliated with an appropriate government agency in Washington;[26] and Albert Ebert, Lloyd's pharmaceutical colleague, spoke for the advantages of Chicago's John Crerar Library, recently formed in 1895.[27] Even as late as 1909, Lloyd was reiterating his desire to place the library elsewhere. "In this connection," he told Kremers, "I will state that I have seen floating paragraphs in the pharmaceutical print, to the effect that it had been decided that the Lloyd Library should remain in Cincinnati. To this I will say that nothing of the kind has been decided. The final resting place of the Library remains to be determined, just as has been the case, from the beginning."[28]

Apparently, Lloyd had grander designs than just relocation. In an extremely interesting letter to James H. Beal in 1910, Lloyd suggested that at "whatever institution the Lloyd Library is located" a "research professorship" ought to be established to conduct a seminar in the history of pharmacy. Indeed, Lloyd suggested the funding of "'Lloyd Lectures' on the history of pharmacy, botany and related sciences."[29]

But Lloyd could not part with his library. He had spent too much time, effort, and money building his collection. Russel Manning, a colleague of Lloyd's, estimated in 1920 that he had expended $100,000 on developing the library.[30] Also, to move the library would mean to separate this valuable research repository from his beloved Eclectic Medical

Institute (after 1910, the Eclectic Medical College). Even as early as 1902, Harvey Wickes Felter noted the close working relationship between the EMI and the Lloyd Library.[31] By the 1930s the EMC was using the library to support its accreditation with the Council of Medical Education, the National Eclectic Medical Association, and the Ohio State Board of Medical Registration and Examination.[32] Helping to support the research needs of the nation's leading eclectic college, the library that John Lloyd and his brother Curtis had amassed could easily stand alone without the help of any established university.

A closer look at the library collection explains why. Curtis and John had carefully selected materials that permitted any researcher to trace out the history of pharmacy and phytomedicine from its earliest beginnings to the present. Attempting to showcase the holdings at the Lloyd Library has been aptly described as "an embarrassment of riches."[33] Yet even the briefest summary, however arbitrary, helps to show the accumulated wealth of material assembled by the brothers. Perhaps the best historical starting point is not the oldest book in the library but an 1875 facsimile of the ancient Egyptian *Papyrus Ebers*, a work dating from about 1550 BC that contains descriptions of seven hundred drugs and more than eight hundred formulas of chiefly botanical origin. This handsomely bound facsimile folio is supplemented by some of pharmacy and botany's rarest treasures, the oldest of which is a 1493 *Mesue vulgare*, or "common book" of remedies written in Italian. Works by Dioscorides (first century AD), the so-called father of our mater medica, Apuleius Barbarus (fifth century AD), the author of the first work to which the term "herbal" was applied, and the four great German patriarchs of botany, Otto Brunfels (?–1534), Jerome Bock (1498–1554), Leonhart Fuchs (1501–1566), and Valerius Cordus (1515–1544), as well as extensive pharmacopeial and dispensatory holdings are just a few highlights of the rare books that Curtis brought back from Europe. In addition, there are scarce volumes representing the development of American pharmacy. Among them are an original 1787 copy of *Materia Medica Americana* by Johann David Schöpf (1752–1800), a book that John Uri Lloyd considered irreplaceable; Benjamin Smith Barton's (1776–1815) important two-volume *Collections for an Essay Towards a Materia Medica of the United States*, a work widely regarded as a predecessor to the *U.S. Pharmacopeia*; and a comprehensive collection of

American pharmacopeial literature that includes the very first work of
its kind in the new nation, the *Pharmacopoeia of the Massachusetts Medical
Society* (1808). When these plus the thousands of other volumes of historical interest are added to contemporaneous monographs and periodicals, it is easy to see why Lloyd had been besieged by university
scholars, provosts, deans, and presidents asking for his library. This was a
ready-made research collection in pharmacy and botany that was not
only historically based but also full of current materials.

Given the priceless character of the library, Lloyd was understandably cautious and somewhat proprietary with his collection. Even
the circulation procedures established at the library show a certain—indeed justifiable—reluctance to adopt a liberal lending policy. The books
at the Lloyd Library were expensive to obtain, and their replacement
(where possible) would have proven too costly both in time and dollars
for them to be loaned out to anyone who just walked through the doors.
By the 1920s the library lending policy was simple and succinct:

RULES FOR OBTAINING BOOKS
The Lloyd Library will loan books only to some other established library, and not to an individual. Books will be sent
on request, by express only; charges to be paid by the recipient.
They should be returned within a reasonable time by express prepaid or registered mail. No books should be entrusted
to the open mails.
Lloyd Library[34]

As the collection grew in strength, Lloyd eventually attempted to
use his library to exert institutional influence in the profession at large.
Some of his efforts were more successful than others. Although his own
writings and reprintings of important pharmaceutical works will be
discussed in the next chapter, it should be noted that the Bulletins of
the Lloyd Library of Botany, Pharmacy and Materia Medica, published
from 1900 to 1936, made important contributions to the literature. John
was also querying members of the APhA about the possibility of using
the Lloyd Library to store the association's archives and to distribute its
publications. The substance of the proposition was that the library would
"take charge of all the publications issued by your society in annual

form and will attend to the addressing and distributing to your members as well as the exchange list." In addition, Lloyd proposed to "take charge of the present stock of back numbers of the Proceedings." Along with these back issues, the library would also become the repository of future issues as they became available, and it would assume all expenses associated with the housing and distribution of these materials, except for mail charges.

Lloyd's offer was referred to the Committee on Publications, whose response was less than enthusiastic. The general feeling was that too many strings were attached; the committee was especially troubled by the loss of ownership of their own publications. "If we ever intend to have a permanent library," the committee concluded, "it would seem better to keep control of all periodicals and text books received. . . . The offer of the Lloyd Library to loan exchanges can doubtless be duplicated elsewhere. Possibly, the St. Louis Library, or the College of Physicians of Philadelphia, or the College of Physicians and Surgeons of New York might be willing to cooperate with the A. Ph. A. in this respect."[35]

The decision was wise for both concerned. From the APhA's perspective, permitting the Lloyd Library to assume so much control over publications bearing its name seems counterproductive; from the Lloyd Library's perspective, the duties of distribution and management of serials (to say nothing of housing back issues) would certainly have diverted valuable dollars and human resources away from the very thing that the library had always done best: develop its own unique collection.

Taken as a whole, however, the Lloyd Library had already gained considerable prestige. Its publications were well known and widely distributed, and the library could count scholars from around the world as its valued patrons. The Lloyds recognized the value of their library and worked to ensure that some provision be made for its future. Here, Curtis played an important part.[36] On February 2, 1917, he established a trust leaving his estate to the care and maintenance of the Lloyd Library.[37]

The question, then, naturally arises: Who really founded the Lloyd Library? On paper the founder is clearly Curtis. He established the trust without which there would be no library today. Curtis also deserves credit for stocking the shelves with expert care and attention; few institutions had amassed so rare and valuable a collection in so relatively few years as had the Lloyd Library. Yet it must be remembered that Curtis's endowment (important though it is) merely guaranteed in perpetuity what was already established legally. In two articles of incorporation with the state of Ohio dated March 25, 1898, and revised November 29, 1907, the mission of the library set forth was "to collect and maintain a library of botanical, medical, pharmaceutical, and scientific books and periodicals and works of allied sciences. . . ."[38] The signatories on both documents, interestingly, included both John Uri and Curtis Gates Lloyd as well as key members of the Eclectic Medical Institute.

Although Curtis played a large and important part in developing the library through his book acquisitions and eventual endowment, John was clearly the funding source for most of the library's ongoing activities during the brothers' lifetimes. From his eclectic preparations to his royalties for *Stringtown*, John was the fuel behind Curtis's book-buying fire. In addition, John himself frequently suggested titles, and with Curtis in Europe much of the time, it was the patriarch of the family who watched over the collection and its management. Despite Curtis's ostensible role, John's hand was in virtually every aspect of the library's operations, even if he did refer particular items of the library to his brother. The few extant letters between John and his brother concerning the library show that Curtis at times needed to be prodded into action. One interesting example concerns the acquisition of the personal papers of Dr. James Pattison Walker (1821–1906), an eclectic surgeon general of the British army. While the library did eventually obtain the materials, it was not without insistent reminders from John.[39] In August 1906, John wrote to Curtis about Walker's bequest of his papers to the Lloyd Library, imploring him, "Please do not delay attending to the matter. It is important." Five months later, John again wrote, "Attend to the Walker bequest. I have heard nothing from it and am being constantly asked questions regarding the condition in which the donation is and when it will be received."[40]

An interesting observation was made by Martin Fischer, a physician and professor of physiology at the University of Cincinnati, who knew all the Lloyds quite well: "To know a man you must see him at his work. To do this in the case of John Uri Lloyd you amble down a quiet side street in Cincinnati and find the pharmaceutical manufacturing concern of Lloyd Brothers: three of them, one of whom seems to watch over the more impractical two, a second who is constantly at molds and never at business, and the third who is the subject of this sketch."[41] There was Nelson Ashley, quiet and hard-working, tending to day-to-day operations, and along with John, constantly researching and testing out new processes and methods; and then there was Curtis, "never at business." There is considerable evidence that the youngest brother, though a devoted mycologist and an avid, expert book-buyer, spent considerable time at play. File after file of Curtis's correspondence contains the letters of women hopeful of catching this wealthy and eligible bachelor. If the sheer number of letters are any indication, the youngest of the Lloyd brothers seemed to enjoy the chase. Fannie, Clara, Lizzie, Katie, Nellie, Mary, Bertha, Anna, Alice, Lulu, Sally, and Minnie were all favorite correspondents with Curtis. To an English woman named Ester Walker, he wrote under the alias Jack H. Hart.[42]

The point of all this is that between Curtis's travels, his mycological pursuits, and his womanizing, little time was left for the library. True, Curtis oversaw certain aspects of library operations (especially building and collection development), but it was John who managed *and* funded the growing institution. The motivations and private intentions of a family's financial affairs are seldom expressed in permanent records, although it is probably no coincidence that the establishment of the trust fund to perpetuate the Lloyd Library was placed in the hands of the one brother without heirs, thus protecting the will and bequest from any possible litigation. This is not to suggest that Curtis did not want to endow the library or that he accepted it only grudgingly, only that each of the brothers was certainly in agreement with a plan that provided legal protections for a bequest and that allowed monies to be quietly funneled into Curtis's account for the library's future.

Besides this is the fact that both his brothers died at least ten years before John (Ashley on January 27, 1925; Curtis on November 11, 1926). This left John in control over library affairs until his own death years later. During this period, the disposition of the library even with a trust in force was at the eldest brother's sole discretion. The library continued to grow, and the remaining Lloyd was still constantly promoting and enlarging the collection as he had from the beginning. In 1928 it was John who published Caswell Mayo's extensive history of the library as issue number 28 of his Bulletin. Even in his later correspondence with

Edward Kremers, the aging Lloyd was still concerned with acquiring materials and making sure that the library got its due recognition.

Whatever else may be said of the respective brothers' roles in assuring the availability of this unique collection for future generations, because of John's crucial influence over funding *and* operations, it is safe to say that the library represents John Lloyd's most lasting and significant contribution to American scholarship. Not only did he leave behind one of the finest collections in its several fields, he also established the library as an ongoing publication arm of his lifelong interest in phytomedicine. Although the library ceased publication of its Bulletin with John Lloyd's death in 1936, by 1938 it was distributing copies of its *Lloydia* to about twelve hundred colleges and universities across the country. For the next twenty years, this refereed journal in pharmacognosy was edited by Theodore Just (1904–1960), a research associate at Northwestern University and lecturer in botany at the University of Chicago. In 1960 the editorial chair was assumed by Arthur Schwarting of the University of Connecticut's School of Pharmacy. In 1961 the journal became a joint publication of the American Society of Pharmacognosy (ASP) and the Lloyd Library and Museum. Changing its name to the *Journal of Natural Products* in 1979, it is still issued with the support of the Lloyd Library, the ASP, and most recently, the American Chemical Society.

Besides the publications produced by the library, there is the collection itself. It is in every respect the lasting reflection of Lloyd's interests and work. Its substantial archives comprise seventeen different collections, including not only the Lloyd brothers' papers but also drug price lists; the botanical research papers of Forest B. H. Brown and Eileen MacFarlane; a collection of pamphlets, announcements, and fliers of approximately eighty U.S. schools of pharmacy; a horticulture collection; and all the extant records of the Eclectic Medical College. Having long since outgrown the Court Street facility, the Lloyd Library of today resides in a 1970 building located at 917 Plum Street (actually the same lot as the 1908 building). Housing some two hundred thousand volumes and with approximately four hundred active journal titles in pharmacy, botany, and phytomedicine, the library has been recognized through the years by noted authorities as a leading research institution in the United States.[43]

This is precisely as John Uri Lloyd would have wanted it, and nowhere is his presence felt more strongly than at the library he founded. The library today reflects the Lloyd brothers as they were in life. Silent and removed from the academic concerns of his other two brothers is Nelson Ashley, his memory preserved only in a few photographs and general biographical pieces written years ago.[44] Yet through those few sketches emerges a man of diligence and business acumen. Given all of John's innovations in pharmacy, it was surely Nelson who managed the Lloyd Brothers firm and made it a financial success. Then there is Curtis. Works of purely botanical interest (especially mycology) represent the interests of the youngest Lloyd, including his *Mycological Writings* series published by the library. There are also extensive photographs taken by this insatiable globe-trotter. Glass negatives and finished prints of Samoa, Mexico, the West Indies, Italy, and Egypt chronicle Curtis's travels. Finally, there is John. The pharmacy holdings, the works on vegetable materia medica, the medicinal plant and ethnobotanical literature, even materials on Kentucky folklore all bear the unmistakable stamp of the senior Lloyd brother.

The Lloyd Library stands as a monument to John Uri Lloyd. "Ah! this antique library is not as a church graveyard," he once wrote, "it is also a mansion to the living. These alcoves are trysting places for elemental shades. Essences of disenthralled minds meet here and revel. Thoughts of the past take shape and live in this atmosphere. . . . I sit in such a weird library and meditate. The shades of grim authors whisper in my ear, skeleton forms oppose my own, and phantoms possess the gloomy alcoves of the library I am building."[45] His writings and the extant records bearing his name are far from the opaque phantasmagoria depicted in these Etidorhpian images. In his published works and in the records of the EMI, Lloyd comes into sharpest focus. His teaching, his textbooks, and his scientific treatises show John Uri Lloyd's relentless investigation and advocacy of phytomedicine that presage today's popular interest in naturopathic healing and alternative medicine. If the figure of Lloyd has any lasting relevance to American science, he must be seen not only as the founder of an outstanding specialized library but also as a contributor to that institution.

7

Lloyd as Scholar

Under the general rubric of scholarship belong John Uri Lloyd's scientific writing, teaching, and academic affiliations. At first glance, adequately covering the subject would appear to be a daunting task. Lloyd wrote by one estimate some five thousand articles in the journals of the day. In Lloyd's teaching and academic connections, there are only institutional records and the occasional reminiscences of students on which to rely. Thus, one must do a considerable amount of spade work to evaluate Lloyd's scholarship. Nevertheless, these problems *are* surmountable.

An assessment of Lloyd's scientific writing becomes more manageable when it is categorized. To begin with, all of his articles may be placed within five broad classes: (1) research papers; (2) extended treatises, including monographs and other collaborative works; (3) introductory papers; (4) editorials; and (5) polemical pieces. The first group represents some of Lloyd's most important work, much of which has been discussed in chapter 5. It includes his three Ebert Prize winners, his other articles on percolation techniques and precipitates, and his research on hydrous aluminum silicate (Lloyd's reagent). The second group stands very nearly equal in importance to the first category. This includes: his textbook *The Chemistry of Medicines* (1st ed., 1881); his book on elixirs (1st ed., 1883); his *References to Capillarity* (1902); his treatise *The Eclectic Alkaloids* (1910); his *Origin and History of All the Pharmacopeial Vegetable Drugs* (1921); and his coauthored works with Curtis Lloyd, John King, Harvey Wickes Felter, and Finley Ellingwood. The third category of writing comprises introductory articles. These are uneven in quality: The worst of these are ruminations on a variety of subjects characterized by imprecise terminology and solecistic prose; the best show the thought processes of an inventive and innovative mind heading toward further investigations, samples of which would include "To What Do Our Plants Owe Their Value?," "Pharmaceutical Trifles," and "Polypharmacy." Lloyd's editorials, the fourth category of writings, often reveal the important medical and pharmaceutical issues of the day and for this reason are valuable primary resources for the historian, but they hardly rank with the first three groups of writings just outlined. Finally, there are Lloyd's polemics. These are numerous and represent his all too frequent exercises in promoting, defending, and otherwise expounding upon eclecticism and sectarian medicine in general.

Grouped in this manner, those writings worthy of further analysis and comment can be vastly reduced. When his penchant for recycling is also taken into account (Lloyd tended to submit essentially the same article to different journals under slightly altered titles), his truly significant publications can be reduced to a much more manageable number (see appendix 4). This massive paring down underscores a very accurate observation made by historian Glenn Sonnedecker: "Lloyd exemplifies a man who wrote too much and too often to meet the exigency of a particular occasion or invitation."[1] This should be borne in mind by anyone who would seek to comprehensively examine Lloyd's scholarly contributions.

At its worst, Lloyd's writing is vague, undisciplined, and idiosyncratic. His tendency to mount the soapbox and expound on topics he was ill-equipped to handle can make Lloyd appear dilettantish and indiscriminate as an author. Those who plod through his voluminous contributions to the *Eclectic Medical Journal*, for example, would be struck by the sometimes curious and eccentric topics that motivated his pen. There is his "Leisure Hours," in which Lloyd proposes to tell other members of his profession (including physicians) how they should be spending their spare time, an impertinent exercise for *anyone*, much less a twenty-nine-year-old; or his "Organized Water as Food" in which he rambles on about everything from soup to jelly fish and winds up speculating about "vitalized water molecules" as "rational food products"; then there is "The Ocean of Vitality and Reservoir of Life," an odd and disjointed fragment from a lecture—introducing, of all things, the subject of vegetation, in which he bounds from chemistry to cosmology to "ask how beginless *[sic]* time commences and passes into time's everlastingness."[2] These articles are clearly misrepresentations of Lloyd's more serious scholarship. They are pointed out to show that, rather than becoming awed by his prolific publication record, the focus needs to be kept narrow and upon those things that reflect Lloyd at his best: his work in medicinal plants, materia medica, chemistry, and pharmacy.

Lloyd gives the historian some help here. In an interesting essay published in 1925, he reflected upon those early works that led him toward fruitful investigations.[3] After recounting his efforts to assist John King in his work on an eclectic pharmacopeia, Lloyd pointed to an 1874 essay titled "To What Do Our Medicinal Plants Owe Their Value?" as directing him away from the old "conglomerate preparations" to "consider individual plants of the vegetable materia medica and to study them severally for the purpose of differentiating between constituents desirable in specifically applied directions, and those undesirable." Noting that earlier authors (eclectic and other American writers) tended to discuss the medicinal properties of a given plant rather vaguely, Lloyd called for a more rigorous and systematic examination of a plant's chemical constituents:

> Chemistry has shown us that every plant contains a number of distinct organic principles, and practice constantly demonstrates that results entirely different are produced upon our organisms by the same plant, and from this we may infer that each of the isolated organic principles chemistry proves exists within the plant, possesses the property of exerting an influence upon our system, or portions of the same, peculiar to that distinct substance; and that although nature has harmonized these principles in the economy of the plant so as to make them necessary to the existence of the plant, yet upon man they produce effects as different as though each were obtained from a separate source.
>
> Now is it desirable to throw the entire system out of order when we wish to produce the specific effect of some particular principle contained within a plant? Would it not be better to isolate the several antagonistic medicinal substances, so as to

produce singly, and at option, the results that are collectively obtained when the crude plant or part of the same is administered?[4]

Most Europeans had already discovered this,[5] but in the context of American research (and particularly with native American plants), Lloyd's insistence upon a more systematic approach to these investigations was one of the most comprehensive and sophisticated calls on this side of the Atlantic. Indeed, this essay sets the tone and substance of Lloyd's work in pharmaceutical chemistry for the remainder of his professional career. Emanating directly from this desire to systematically isolate phytochemical constituents was a series of nine essays published from early 1875 through the summer of 1876 collectively titled "Pharmaceutical Chemistry." It is not surprising that Lloyd singled these articles out fifty years later as important, for they were preliminary to his book-length treatment, *The Chemistry of Medicines*. Widely regarded as one of the first American textbooks on pharmaceutical chemistry written by a pharmacist, Lloyd's book was popular in the classroom, as attested to in its eight editions from 1881 to 1897.[6] His interest in the chemistry of medicinal plants ultimately yielded an Ebert Prize in 1891 for his "Schemes of Assaying."

Also important for Lloyd was his short essay, "Pharmaceutical Trifles." In this article he first revealed his interest in the principles underlying tinctures, fluidextracts, precipitates, and filtration. "Did you ever have a turbid mixture which you wished to filter, but could not, for seemingly from pure perverseness it *would not filter?*," he asked. "Did you ever come across a preparation that should have been clear, but instead was opalescent, or I rather should say translucent? and when an attempt was made to correct the imperfection by filtration, did you discover it could not be done, and that although the mixture was passing rapidly through the paper, it *would not improve*, but even though it were filtered over and over, time and again, it would still remain as objectionable as at the commencement?"[7] His efforts at solving these vexing questions brought him national and international recognition. Through his "Precipitates in Fluid Extracts" published six years later, he earned his first Ebert Prize from the American Pharmaceutical Association, and in 1916 his work was translated in the important German journal *Kolloidchemische Beihefte.*

The final essay singled out by Lloyd as significant was an 1887 article titled "Polypharmacy." Here he chided those pharmacists who made unsystematic hodgepodges of vegetable products. This practice was rampant in the 1880s and stemmed from a long-standing "more is better" approach to therapeutics. Typical were odd combinations of mineral and botanical substances like "Tully's Mixture of Iron and Conium [i.e., poison hemlock!]," which *also* included tolu, cinnamon, cassia, and gaultheria; and "De Vigo's Mercurial Plaster," which contained a dozen different ingredients.[8] Quoting the eclectic physician Andrew Jackson Howe (1825–1892) who called this polypharmacy a "prolix combination of drugs [that] is sure to embarrass and antagonize," Lloyd complained against "the mixing up of a promiscuous mess of inert drugs with one that is valuable as a remedy. In each instance the impurities—dirt, if you choose to call it dirt—not only are of no use, but interfere with the action of the valuable ingredient."[9] Lloyd's call for more precisely compounded preparations based upon the careful analysis of each chemical agent undoubtedly recalled to his mind the vast strides that had been made in legislating uniform drug standards nationwide by 1925. Although his polypharmacy did not launch him into award-winning studies, it typifies his efforts at promoting high-quality pharmaceuticals tested for efficacy and purity—efforts that included his strong support of the Pure Food and Drug Act of 1906.[10]

Taken as a whole, his "To What Do Our Medicinal Plants Owe Their Value?," "Pharmaceutical Trifles," and "Polypharmacy" may be considered some of Lloyd's best writing of a preliminary or introductory nature. Objective and concise, these articles were outgrowths of his ongoing lab work. They are important in that they point the way to his more extensive research in pharmacy, and they demonstrate that Lloyd's apparent wizardry was not the product of brilliant flashes of insight but rather the product of long, laborious trial and error, spurred on by perseverance and an insatiable curiosity.

The first book-length study by John Uri Lloyd was his *Supplement to the American Dispensatory,* a 202-page work that he completed in 1880 with his mentor John King. This was a natural extension of his earlier efforts at assisting King with the eclectic pharmacopeia project. By 1880 *King's American Dispensatory* was in its twelfth edition, and by that time it had become the "standard authority on vegetable remedies" for America's eclectic practitioners.[11] Lloyd's coauthorship with one of the EMI's outstanding luminaries shows not only that Lloyd had gained admittance to eclecticism's inner sanctum but that he was now a fully recognized member of its elite.

In order to appreciate the importance of this *Supplement*, it is necessary to understand the place of the *American Dispensatory* in eclectic literature. This reference tool was *not* designed to supplant the *USP* or *USD*. From the very beginning, King adhered to those remedies and preparations "recognized by the United States Pharmacopeia,"[12] but he did add those botanicals and other agents generally used by eclectics that were not included among these regular pharmaceutical sources. In effect, the *American Dispensatory* was designed to be its own official guide for the eclectic practitioner and compounder of eclectic preparations. On June 19, 1879, at the annual meeting of the National Eclectic Medical Association held in Chicago, Secretary Alexander Wilder recorded the following: "*Resolved*, That this Association adopt *The American Dispensatory* as its *standard authority*."[13]

To assist in developing future editions of this important eclectic work, King called upon John Lloyd as coauthor. Referring to him as "a theoretical and practical chemist and pharmacist, well known to the pharmacists of this country," King indicated that "this arrangement will continue through subsequent editions."[14] Indeed it did, even extending beyond King's death in 1893 to include Lloyd's collaborative editions with fellow eclectic Harvey Wickes Felter. It was in this 1880 *Supplement* that this long and fruitful alliance began.

King's selection of Lloyd as a collaborator was a wise one. The *American Dispensatory* could not be created in a vacuum; what was needed to make this official eclectic reference manual truly useful was a strong link with the regular pharmaceutical community. This he found in Lloyd, who had, in fact, been quietly assisting Charles Rice in his extremely important sixth revision of the *USP*. In an interesting and revelatory letter to Edward Kremers some forty years later, Lloyd recounted his entry into the pharmacopeial revision process:

When Dr. Rice was made Chairman of the Committee of Rivision [sic] for the Pharmacopeia of the U.S., the committee awarded him to do the work was not a very satisfactory one in some directions. Professor J. F. Judge, of Cincinnati, was one of that Committee, and to Dr. Judge was given by Dr. Rice a phase of the work embracing solubilities and other problems connected therewith. Professor Judge did absolutely nothing. Rice had relied upon him, and as Dr. Rice wrote me when he asked me to take charge of that work, Judge had ceased replying to his letters. I took upon myself the research Rice wanted done, on condition that the name of Professor Judge should stand, and that I should be unmentioned therein. In this Dr. Rice reluctantly agreed.

If you will take that copy of the Pharmacopeia, I believe if memory serves me aright, you will find Judge's name carried throughout as one of the Revision Committee, and you will find simply in Dr. Rice's introduction, credit given to me for assistance when called upon. This memory only, but memory in cases like this is likely to be pretty nearly correct.

Now you might ask, in what particular direction should I be credited in this work. I will tell you. Judge was one of the men who had banded together to destroy me personally, because of my connection with Eclecticism. He had been professor of chemistry in the Eclectic Medical College [i.e., Institute], and he resigned, making public statement that was not complimentary to the school. I took his place, and made a success in a direction where as a teacher he had failed. This led to a personal enmity toward me, which I never in any wise merited, and never noticed by any return whatever. When Judge failed in business he opened up a little store in an insignificant part of Cincinnati. He was absolutely out of money, and could not establish himself. I gave him a stock of goods, full well knowing that they would be lost, and they were. This incident or some other incident connected therewith came to the ears of Dr. Rice, who wrote me a letter concerning the manner in which I had, in a way almost unprecedented, behaved throughout the whole affair, he being aware that Judge was one of the men who had attempted to have me expelled from the American Pharmaceutical Association because of an incident in which I gave the world the botanical names of certain drugs that had been distributed under names unknown to science, their true botanical names not being given, thus disturbing a business that felt aggrieved over the intrusion I had made in that direction.[15]

True to the agreement, the name of John F. Judge, M.D., a member of the Committee of Revision for the sixth decennial revision of the *USP*, was retained in the preface to that work, with John Uri Lloyd's "valuable assistance" acknowledged by his good friend and chair of the committee, Charles Rice.[16] Lloyd's version of his role in the revision process is believable, for his relationship with Rice clearly grew stronger during this period. It is obvious that Lloyd's assistance with Rice's pharmacopeial work blossomed into a friendship that lasted until the death of the great Bellevue Hospital pharmacist in 1901.[17]

Lloyd could not have entered the revision process at a more auspicious time. The sixth revision of the *USP* reflected huge changes in U.S. officinals. In this edition, spearheaded by Charles Rice, 229 outdated remedies were dropped from the *USP* while 236 new preparations were added.[18] Considered by historians of pharmacy as the most sweeping pharmacopeial revision ever, the 1880 *USP* established the format and focus of this pharmaceutical reference work for years to come. As Glenn Sonnedecker explains:

> Any pharmacist who holds this book in his hands and compares it with its predecessor will recognize the advent of the modern *Pharmacopeia of the United States* and will appreciate why this edition signaled a fundamental advance in drug standards for the American health professions and the public.
>
> The new *Pharmacopeia* turned more sharply away from the outworn concept of the community pharmacy as the place of manufacture of most of the pharmaceutical preparations. Instead it tried to establish in the pharmacy another kind of responsibility: examination of medicinal substances by the pharmacist as a check on quality. Casual mention of a few tests was

replaced with detailed tests for identifying and determining the purity of many of the drugs. Detailed processes for assaying the alkaloids appeared for the first time. Drugs from the vegetable and mineral kingdoms were more meaningfully described as to physical characteristics and, where possible, chemical properties. Symbolic formulas and molecular weights were introduced.[19]

Thus, John Uri Lloyd's assistance in Rice's pharmacopeial work placed the eclectic pharmacist on the cutting edge of his discipline.

Lloyd's *Supplement to the American Dispensatory* is divided into two parts: Part one (the vast majority of the book) covers "Materia Medica"; part two deals with "Pharmacy and Pharmacopeia." From acidum chrysophanicum to verbesina, the alphabetical entries include pertinent information regarding formulas, preparation, history, properties, and uses of each product. The second section on pharmacy includes articles on a variety of fluidextracts. The book concludes with an appendix of "several articles that have been recently introduced (or re-introduced) to the profession, some of which, undoubtedly, possess valuable therapeutical properties."

Initially offered for the first three months at $2 per copy, and afterward sold only with the *Dispensatory* for a total cost of $10, the *Supplement*'s reception by the eclectic community was expectedly favorable. "We have looked over the proof sheets," said the *Eclectic Medical Journal* in June of 1880, "and we think the work well done, and that our readers will do well to procure this volume, if they have the *Dispensatory*, or order the new edition of the *Dispensatory* with the supplement. Much care has been used in describing the new chemicals, and indeed in every part," concluded the journal, "and this volume will supply our wants for several years, or until an entirely new edition of the *Dispensatory* is called for."[20] Yet it would be wrong to conclude that this eclectic reference work was valued only by the sectarian community. The *American Journal of Pharmacy* published by the Philadelphia College of Pharmacy—that bedrock of pharmaceutical orthodoxy—called the *Supplement* "one that should be in the library of every pharmacist who would keep himself well informed upon the new remedies which have been introduced."[21]

As important as the *Supplement* was to Lloyd's career, the following year would witness the publication of an even more important work: his book *The Chemistry of Medicines*. Early in 1881, the *Druggists Circular* announced that the volume "is soon to be published." Teasing the readers, the *Circular* suggested that, "judging from some of the advance sheets the treatise will be quite an instructive one."[22] With the release of the book one month later, the *Circular* called this compendium of medicinal chemistry selling for $2.75, "a valuable addition to the library, useful for all, and almost indispensable to the student in medicine and pharmacy."[23] The *Eclectic Medical Journal* had high praise for this production from one of their own. The journal's detailed description of the work shows its value as a textbook:

> The new work upon chemistry is now before us. Instead of three hundred pages as calculated, it contains four hundred and fifty. It opens with a description of apparatus to be used by students, and a figure of each piece mentioned is introduced. This is a valuable point for beginners. The second section gives the "theory of chemistry," in simple language, and we notice that the meaning of about every term employed by chemists is made plain. The non-metallic elements are noticed, and under each element all of the compounds of that element which are used in medicine. The acids are considered under hydrogen, acids being *salts* of hydrogen. The metals now follow, and after a description of each metal, the compounds of that element which are used in medicine are separately considered. Part second of the work is devoted to *organic chemistry*, all alkaloids, resins, ethers, glucosides, etc., being carefully treated. The book ends with a chapter on urinary analysis, in which plain directions are given for examination of urine. These processes are brief, but so plain that any one can follow and be sure of accuracy. Physicians, as a rule, have not the time to "boil down" the large works upon urinary analysis, and Mr. Lloyd saves them this trouble. Practical processes are given for making most chemicals. Adulterations have been especially considered, and tests for them given. Antidotes to poisons are always named and the treatment for poisoning. Every student of medicine should obtain this book.[24]

Other journals outside the eclectic fold found Lloyd's *Chemistry of Medicines* equally praiseworthy. The *Druggist* concluded that the book had "special value to pharmaceutical students," while others called the work "useful" with many "practical hints" in employing the principles of chemistry to medicinal ends.[25] The great favor that greeted Lloyd's first solo effort at writing a book-length treatise yielded results. The Robert Clarke company was completely exhausted of copies within a month of its release, prompting the second of what would become eight editions of the work.

In the midst of success for *The Chemistry of Medicines*, Lloyd released the first of what would be three editions of his book on elixirs (see appendix 4 for details). These hydroalcoholic products had become quite popular in the United States following the Civil War, even becoming a faddish rage by the 1870s.[26] Elixirs were defined by Remington as "aromatic, sweetened, spirituous preparations containing small quantities of active medicinal substances,"[27] and this broad, vague definition pointed to the fundamental problem with all elixirs: Most lacked official status, and no generally accepted standards of quality were available to pharmacists. The hope of many pharmacists that the "elixir swindle" would die a natural death proved unrealistic as the market was flooded with an array of proprietary elixir "remedies" of dubious efficacy. Historian Gregory J. Higby summarizes the dilemma:

> Pharmacists were in a bind, with two great difficulties to solve: How to design elixir formulas that were both "elegant" and potent; and, most importantly, how to convince physicians to prescribe those formulas rather than ready-made elixirs. Over two hundred pharmacists who were not members of the APhA wrote to its secretary, John Maish, asking for the Association's elixir formulas that had been published in a sixteen page pamphlet in 1873. Many wrote back in disappointment at the poor quality of the elixirs produced according to those directions. One member commented that he had "heard considerable ridicule thrown upon the Association in consequence of those formulas" and urged that the Association avoid endorsing specific recipes. Apparently frustrated by the increasing growth in

the number and variety of elixirs and similar preparations, the APhA turned away from the subject for a few years.[28]

Lloyd was very familiar with the elixir problem. Charles Rice, chair of the *USP* revision committee, had privately consulted him in response to Edward R. Squibb's adamant opposition to the acceptance of some elixir formulas into the 1880 decennial revision of the *USP* as "unscientific, unprofessional, illogical conglomerates."[29] Lloyd pointed out that the eclectics, mainly through the writings of John Milton Scudder, were also opposed to these dosage forms. Despite this, Lloyd told Rice "that in my opinion it is the duty of the pharmacopeia to furnish processes for making shop preparations and establishing quantities that would give informal doses to compounds such as were the principle elixirs then in commerce; that I believed, and agreed exactly with Dr. Squibb in that it was a fad, but differed with him in that of the province occupied by the pharmacopeia and its duty to the professions of pharmacy and medicine. My answer seemed to please Dr. Rice."

In some senses, Lloyd's discussion with the revision committee chair is a bit misleading. The question was not really the acceptance of elixirs into the pharmacopeia as a class of remedies: For example, an old preparation called "elixir of vitriol" had been listed in the *USP* as early as 1820.[30] But elixirs in general were never truly part of the U.S. pharmacopeia—certainly *not* the proprietary elixirs flooding the market following the Civil War. Elixirs did not figure prominently in *any* edition of the *USP*, and those that were included were largely intended to be used as vehicles through which active agents could be administered rather than as medications themselves.[31] Despite his advice to Rice, Lloyd recognized that the USP was not the immediate answer to the elixir problem: Something was needed *now*. Thus prompted by his private exchange with Rice, Lloyd wrote *Elixirs: Their History, Formulae, and Methods of Preparation* in 1883, "the main object of that book," he told Kremers years later, "being to put into the hands of pharmacists and physicians processes by which trade elixirs could be paralleled by the apothecary, and it will be noted, if you will refer to Lloyd's Elixir Book, that Dr. Rice wrote the introduction thereof, giving the derivation of the word 'elixir' and its application in pharmacy gone by."

Having himself been besieged by requests for reliable elixir formulas, John Maisch, editor of the *American Journal of Pharmacy*, was undoubtedly relieved to see at last a book-length treatment on this topic. With 283 elixir formulas, it immediately became *the* reference work to consult on this class of preparations. Predictably, Maisch's journal gratefully acknowledged Lloyd's contribution to this controversial dosage form:

> It was not an easy task for the author to collect and critically examine the numerous formulas for elixirs which are scattered through the journals and other publications during the past 24 years; but it has been accomplished, and the author's own experience with this class of preparations has been added, introducing improvements and practical useful suggestions. Of the old-fashioned elixirs, all the important ones have been selected, mostly with the more or less modernized formulas.
>
> The book gives full, and what is better, reliable information about the numerous elixirs more or less in use. . . . [32]

Elixirs was long overdue. Lloyd was a pragmatist when it came to issues of this sort. The profession could not simply wish the "elixir craze" away and ignore it, nor could pharmacists afford to belligerently oppose elixirs as Squibb had. Lloyd's general support of this dosage form made financial *and* professional sense. "At the present time there undoubtedly exists a demand for this class of preparations," wrote Lloyd in his preface, "and, in order to improve, as well as retain, their legitimate trade, our pharmacists are, in a measure, compelled to dispense them, as they do not desire to displease their medical patrons by any indications of what might be considered an offensive dictation. Such being the case, and, as a large number of the pharmacists of this country are not possessors of the past numbers of pharmaceutical journals, we have been induced to produce this little book."[33] Approaching elixirs objectively, Lloyd subjected this dosage form to careful analysis along with some "friendly pruning."

In the end, it was not the pharmacopeia that would be the mainstay of the elixir. The solution to the problem was to incorporate these largely unofficial preparations into a national formulary. A large step in that direction was taken at the suggestion of Samuel Bendiner, who proposed a formulary of unofficial preparations for New York and vicinity. The resulting *New York and Brooklyn Formulary* (1884) helped to create a foundation from which Rice could put together the first edition of *The National Formulary of Unofficinal Preparations* (often referred to simply as the *NF*) in 1888.[34] Here the elixir appeared in force—eighty-six strong.[35]

Lloyd's *Elixirs*, plus the role he played in Rice's private consultations on this issue, was an important factor in creating the impetus for a formulary of national proportions. This represents no small contribution to American pharmacy. Higby has stated that "the NF was devised to treat an ailment that was weakening American pharmacy and threatening its professional life—the rise of the manufacturing of ready-made medicines and proprietary drugs for prescriptions. American pharmacy was going through a transitional phase from an older model of professionalism based on individual demonstration of skill and honesty to the modern form of professionalism based on paper credentials such as diplomas and registration certificates. For the professionally-minded APhA member of 1888, in-house manufacture of preparations was the prime foundation of their professionalism."[36] In this sense, Higby has called the development of the *NF* "a turning point for American pharmacy." If so, Lloyd clearly helped to steer his profession toward modernity as Rice's confidant and as the author of *Elixirs*. Indeed, *The National Formulary* has acknowledged Lloyd's book along with the *New York and Brooklyn Formulary* as the "decided stimulus" for an authoritative compendium of unofficial preparations in the United States.[37]

Shortly after the appearance of his elixir book, John Lloyd announced an ambitious collaborative project with his botanist brother Curtis to produce "not later than April, 1884," a serial publication titled *Drugs and Medicines of North America* to "represent all known researches in this important field."[38] True to their word, the May issue of the *Druggists Circular* carried a laudatory review, noting that, with a subscription price of $1 per year or 30¢ per issue, "Never was a work of such merit offered to the pharmacist on terms so moderate. It ought to find a place in every physician's and druggist's library." The response of other journals were equally favorable.[39]

Price was not the problem, however. Unfortunately, after covering the Ranunculaceae family and an assortment of noteworthy medicinals like lobelia, wild allspice, and cohosh, the plan eventually collapsed under the weight of its own magnitude. The last of a mere two volumes closed the periodical in June of 1887. Yet the Lloyds had made an important effort. Reissued in book form as part of Lloyd Library Bulletin numbers 29–31, the 1930 reprinting had an important foreword by Edward Kremers, which put this aborted but laudable effort into some context:

> The first edition of *Pharmacographia* by Flückiger and Hanbury had appeared in 1874, the second in 1879. While American medicinal plants had by no means been ignored, the rapid development of American vegetable materia medica seemed to call for either a supplement or a treatise of its own. Schoepf, the Hessian army surgeon, after the War of Independence, had explored the North American flora and had written a *Materia Medica Americana* in 1787, reprinted as *Bulletin of the Lloyd Library* in . . . 1903. However, this contained but brief botanical descriptions. Bartram and his students at the University of Pennsylvania had published a number of monographs in which the chemical constituents of the plants as well as their therapeutic action received such consideration as was possible at the time. Maisch, at the Philadelphia College of Pharmacy, had published abstracts from graduation theses in which extraction with selective solvents à la Dragendorff played an important role. The pharmaceutical manufacturers representing the Eclectic School of Medicine had made a specialty of galenicals from American medicinal plants which resulted in the isolation, for the most part in a crude and impure condition, of certain groups of therapeutically active substances, such as the resinoids. It remained, however, for John Uri Lloyd to make an intensive study of a number of plants that had acquired therapeutic significance. In this he was aided by the facilities of a manufacturing laboratory [and his brother Curtis] as contrasted with the meager opportunities, so far as quantity was concerned, of the investigator in the college laboratories.[40]

Although the results fell far short of John Lloyd's grand scheme, others recognized his talents and expertise. When the great European pharmacognosist Friedrich Flückiger came to America in the summer of 1894, he visited Lloyd at his library in Cincinnati and requested that John contribute chapters on American medicinal plants to his *History of Drugs*. Unfortunately, Flückiger died in Geneva shortly thereafter, but not Lloyd's dream of creating a comprehensive reference work on all the American medicinal plants. In many ways, the library that he built represented his continued desire to at least compile the works requisite to this unfinished task, and herein perhaps represents the most significant feature of *Drugs and Medicines of North America*.[41] It might also be stated in passing that the only publication even approaching the scope of Lloyd's unfinished magnum opus was Charles F. Millspaugh's *American Medicinal Plants*.[42] Thorough and richly illustrated as it was, however, even this work could not be called comprehensive.

Following his *Drugs and Medicines of North America*, the other productions from John Uri Lloyd's pen that fit into this genre of book-length treatises and monographs in many ways reflect efforts already initiated. His collaboration with John King continued on *The American Dispensatory*, and after King's death with Harvey Wickes Felter as *King's American Dispensatory*; his *References to Capillarity*, published as Lloyd Library Bulletin number 4 in 1902, examined and synthesized much of his Ebert Prize winning work published as journal articles; his *Eclectic Alkaloids, Resins, Resinoids, Oleo-Resins and Concentrated Principles*, published as Bulletin number 12 in 1910, represents one of Lloyd's best historical efforts in his discussion of the concentration "craze" (see chapter 3 for details); and his contribution to Finley Ellingwood's *American Materia Medica, Therapeutics, and Pharmacognosy* in 1915 and 1919 demonstrates Lloyd's willingness to lend his name and support to the efforts of eclectic colleagues.[43]

One book, however, must still be discussed: his *Origin and History of All the Pharmacopeial Vegetable Drugs* (1921; reprinted 1929). This 449-page treatment of the vegetable products listed in the eighth and ninth decennial revisions of the *USP* is, if nothing else, a testimony to the vitality of the seventy-year-old pharmacist. Lloyd compiled and alphabetically arranged historical data and other information on 168 different plants and discussed their pharmaceutical and ethnobotanical uses, their initial introduction dates into the *USP*, and their official pharmacopeial status. Although the projected continuation by Lloyd's longtime chemist colleague Sigmund Waldbott never resulted in a published second volume on chemical drugs, Lloyd's book stands on its own. By honing in on those representatives of America's vegetable materia medica included in the *USP*, Lloyd's *Origin and History of All the Pharmacopeial Vegetable Drugs* succeeded where his *Drugs and Medicines of North America* had failed. Unlike the massive task of treating thousands of American medicinal plants, this book had a very specific and manageable (albeit challenging) objective. The volume was commissioned by the American Drug Manufacturers' Association as the result of a special meeting of the Committee on Standards and Deteriorations held on March 30, 1917, at New York's Waldorf-Astoria. The committee had a very clear idea of what it wanted: namely, "an historical investigation of the drugs and preparations official in the *Pharmacopeia of the United States*." [44] In 1921 John Uri Lloyd gave the committee a very creditable work. Moreover, pharmacy got a book that has withstood the test of time. At least one contemporary analyst has called it "encyclopedic" and "still useful." Reading this compendium today, the assessment of one historian can still stand unaltered: "If we do not try to judge this volume as history but as the reference intended, it must be admitted, however far the book is from being exhaustive, that scarcely anywhere else in the Americas at this time could the particular combination and dimensions of mind and resources be found to produce such a work." [45]

Having discussed Lloyd's research papers in the previous chapter, plus the most important of his introductory articles and book-length treatises, I must mention his editorial work. As a reprinter of classic works on materia medica through his Reproduction Series of the Lloyd Library Bulletin, Lloyd played the role of editor often introducing works, reformatting them, and getting others (such as Edward Kremers) to add their historical perspectives on the significance of the work at hand. Lloyd's efforts in this regard are valuable contributions to the literature and helped to rescue many a rare and nearly forgotten tome from oblivion.

But Lloyd did not rest with this. When W. C. Cooper, who had originated the *Eclectic Medical Gleaner* in 1894 along with Dr. W. E. Bloyer, resigned his position as editor, the publication was taken over by the

Lloyd Library. In September of 1904, the new editor, Harvey Wickes Felter, released volume 15, number 9, with little noticeable change in style or format. In January of the following year, however, the *Gleaner* took on a new appearance with expanded contents that included John Uri Lloyd as editor of the "Publishers' Department." Although the journal shifted from a monthly to a bimonthly publication beginning in 1905, it showed no lack of energy in promoting the eclectic cause for the next seven years. Felter's resignation from his editorial duties at the close of 1912 prompted the final issue of the *Gleaner*, in which Lloyd wrote a glowing biographical sketch of his friend and colleague. Despite the periodical's comparatively short run, Lloyd's close connections with it provided him with another sounding board—in addition to his frequent contributions in the *Eclectic Medical Journal*—in which to hold forth on a wide variety of topics from drugs in history to adulteration issues, eclecticism, the taste of medicines, and so on. Thus, it might be said that Lloyd's editorial work in some appreciable ways contributed to his polemical writings on a diffused body of subject matter.

Lloyd's writings provide only one dimension of his scholarship, however. Lloyd had strong connections with academia as well. The fact that he actively taught at *both* the Eclectic Medical Institute and, from 1883 to 1887, at the Cincinnati College of Pharmacy is a testimony to the acceptance and esteem for his work across sectarian lines. Despite this fact, the EMI was his true love, and it was to this school that he devoted most of his attentions. Lloyd took over the position of professor of chemistry and pharmacy at the institute from John A. Jeancon (1831–1903), a position he held until receiving emeritus status in 1907. Lloyd also held a variety of positions on the board of trustees, beginning as president with the 1896–1897 academic term and concluding as vice president in 1905.[46] John Uri Lloyd's long and distinguished tenure at the EMI earned him rank as one of the school's "Old Seven"—an august body of eclectic leading lights consisting of John King, John Milton Scudder, Edwin Freeman, Andrew Jackson Howe, John A. Jeancon, and Frederick J. Locke.

While Lloyd became one of the foundational giants at the EMI, his classroom methods, albeit a bit unorthodox, were apparently appreciated by his students. Rolla Thomas, class of 1880 and dean of the EMI and

EMC, fondly remembered his methods. "Some of us were so stupid," he admitted. "And yet with that patience which characterized him at all times, he was able to get some chemistry and pharmacy into the most stupid pupils. A successful teacher must be a good disciplinarian. Yet the Professor never had to enforce discipline."[47] Well, *almost* never. A mere twenty-nine years old and described by himself as a "little runt," Lloyd got wind of a plot to literally toss him out of the classroom on his maiden voyage as professor of chemistry. School hooligans had given the EMI faculty trouble before. Jeancon, Lloyd's immediate predecessor, for example, was remembered by one EMI graduate as a "decided failure" as a disciplinarian and one whose classes were "looked forward to with true delight by the mischief-loving contingent of the students."[48] Therefore, when the diminutive Lloyd made his appearance, class cutups were eager to take advantage of this young fledgling and maintain the tradition of high jinks in the EMI chemistry classes. Proving that classroom disruptions are not simply a present-day phenomenon, Lloyd remembered his very first class:

> The class was immense, several hundred in number. I waited till they all were in the room. I then went in, stepped in front of the table that stood on a little platform and raised my finger, eyeing the class but never looking at the finger. It was a critical moment, that even the leaders of the proposed disturbance appreciated. They began to get quiet; soon I could locate but a little noise, in a group down in the center of the room. I looked directly at the point of disturbance, and pointed my finger at the group. They knew—so did I—that it was whip or be whipped. A profound silence followed. "Listen," was my opening remark. "I am here to teach you chemistry and you are here to learn chemistry. Either you will listen to me this hour through, quiet, or I shall leave the room, never again to come back. You must make your choice now."
>
> After a brief interval I continued: "If there is any man in this room who proposes not to listen after the manner I have mentioned, let him hold up his hand. I want to face him now." Not a hand went up.

"Now," I said, "my friends, there are some rules that I am going to lay down that I propose to follow, and intend that you shall follow. They are as follows:

"First, courteous attention is due, each to the other. I shall give it to you, you must give it to me.

"Second, we have a Board of Trustees in this college. The first man who throws a paper ball across the room will be reported to the Board of Trustees to be expelled for insubordination. Either he will leave the college or the class will get no further instruction from me.

"Third, whoever feels that he must whisper, because of the importance of the subject, may hold up his hand. I will either excuse him from the room, or let him speak aloud so as to instruct us all. I will not only give him a chance to serve his classmates, but myself will listen, and will profit thereby.

"Whoever whistles during a lecture may not get caught, but if he is caught it means report to the Board of Trustees.

"Now I hope we understand each other. The lesson today is introductory chemistry, and tomorrow I shall quiz this class on what is given today."[49]

Lloyd's lectures were usually not so confrontational. Typically, initial lectures to incoming students at the institute were, in the words of one recipient, "studded with good counsel and fatherly advice." Lloyd, no doubt harking back to his own rustic awe of the bustling river town, took special care to warn of Cincinnati's "gilded palaces of vice" and cautioned those from distant locales that their conduct was under constant scrutiny: "I tell you," Lloyd declared, "the very walls will speak!"[50] Having delivered the standard caveats, Lloyd launched into his routine of instruction. Details of his actual classroom materials are lacking due to his habit of lecturing sans notes; but his classes did not lack for substantive content, for he often kept the class late as he touched on various topics old and new to the field of chemistry.[51] Armed only with their required text (Lloyd's own *Chemistry of Medicines*), the young men, hopeful of some day placing M. D. after their names, faced a challenging subject with eclecticism's greatest figure.

Despite the lack of information on Lloyd's lectures, Charles L. Olsen provides a rare and detailed glimpse of Professor Lloyd's physical appearance, classroom demeanor, and personality:

John Uri Lloyd: Small of stature and spare of form; neat as a new pin; unostentatious to an extreme; dressed very plainly but faultlessly, and always with a small nosegay—preferably a delicate little rose—in the button hole of the left lapel of his coat, noiselessly he entered and with a quick, quiet, elastic step reached the platform. He seemed to evince more than an ordinary interest in the welfare of the college. First, he would glance over the bulletin, looking for special announcements, referring to them, if necessary; then he scanned the black board for the outline of the day's lesson (performed by his assistant, Prof. Felter). Now turning to the table near the edge of the platform, on which had been placed the paraphernalia necessary for demonstration, he would first examine the display, closely inspecting everything, to make sure that all needed material for the lesson was on hand, and arranged *just so*. Then, and not before, with an air of readiness, his left arm akimbo—the thumb pointing forward and the index finger downward—he *very lightly* rapped on the table for attention, not with his delicate knuckles, however, but with the back of his hand turned downward he would make the little gold ring, worn on the right ring-finger, do the duty. With head inclined at one angle of about 45°, his mild eyes sweeping over the assembly from right to left, or vise versa, the stereotyped "Ladies and Gentlemen," quickly uttered, meant, "Now, listen to me." And they had to for his was not a stentorian voice.

As all great men are extremists, so Prof. Lloyd was one. In this respect: He would not permit the students to take notes during his lectures. Pencils and notebooks were simply tabooed. To the writer of this, with whom pencil and paper are second nature, such an interdiction seemed a positive hardship.

With Prof. Lloyd there was absolutely nothing fearful, neither in his entrance, his manners or his exit; but as nearly all of his students realized that they were sitting at the feet of a master—one towering head and shoulders above his fellows in the realms of Chemistry and Pharmacy—they paid profound and respectful attention to his utterances. Kind and considerate, and gentle as a maiden he used no force, except the force of reason, in dealing with students; but they invariably yielded to his wish, if even expressed in a whisper. It happened once, and once only, that his patience gave way. For some reason, just at the beginning of a lecture, a ripple of merriment passed over the class, resulting in in-attention. Prof. Lloyd told the students he could not, and if he could, he would not, match his voice nor pit himself against their combined efforts. And this was his punishment: "Prof. Felter will now take you in hand and quiz you during the whole hour." Then, without showing any anger, whatever, expressing the hope that at the next lecture there would be no disturbance of any sort, he took his hat, bowed and left."[52]

Lloyd's method's were designed to keep classroom antics to a minimum and by and large they worked. Yet Lloyd's prohibition of notes and his readiness to give impromptu exams should not suggest that he was a pedagogical martinet. Lloyd was attempting to instill in these budding eclectic physicians the memory of a compounding pharmacist (just as Gordon and Eger had done with him years before). This would serve them well throughout their careers since they would be expected to write prescriptions for their patients. His swift response to any outburst in his classroom was as much intended to instill discipline *within* his students as it was to maintain order in the classroom. Extant examinations for his chemistry classes could hardly be called severe or unfair. They were clearly fashioned to test the bare essentials of the discipline (see appendix 5).

Whether as a writer or a teacher, by the 1890s John Uri Lloyd had established a national reputation as a scholar of merit in chemistry and pharmacy. All of his major works had received highly favorable reviews in the professional literature and by century's end, with the passing of both John King and John Milton Scudder, he was the reigning icon of American eclecticism. While others such as Finley Ellingwood (1852–1920), Harvey Wickes Felter (1865–1927), and Rolla L. Thomas (1857–1932) were prominent within eclectic circles, none of them approached the wide acceptance and acknowledged stature of John Uri Lloyd. In

1895 Lloyd's career would take on added dimensions, for in that year he released his first literary effort, *Etidorhpa*. This odd production of fantastic fiction would launch the first of many novels for the Cincinnati scholar. This leap from pharmacy to literature netted major returns in both dollars and distinction for Lloyd in a whole new sphere. So significant are his efforts in this realm that pharmaceutical historian George Urdang has written: "There are only a few pharmacists who have attained more than local fame in American literature. A thorough and discriminating examination leaves in fact only one member of the profession whose writing was comprehensive and valuable enough to give him a place among American novelists: John Uri Lloyd."[53]

8

Lloyd as Litterateur

The remarkable history of *Etidorhpa, or The End of Earth* began with a small printing by the author in 1895 that was sold only to subscribers, mainly Lloyd's friends and colleagues. Soon thereafter, however, the book was published by the Robert Clarke Company and marketed to the general public.[1] John Uri Lloyd introduced himself to the literary world with a work that at first defied definitive interpretation. Was this work revelatory? Was it prophetic? Was it a dystopian warning or a utopian promise? While it is classed in most modern reference sources as science fiction,[2] the specific genre of this work is not of primary concern. In its century-long history, it has received a variety of labels too many to mention. What it has accomplished is far more interesting: It has garnered a devoted following of readers for more than one hundred years.

Since most readers today are probably unfamiliar with this novel, a brief recounting of the tale seems appropriate. The story is ostensibly about a trip to the inner earth and appears cloaked in mystery, as its lengthy subtitle claims to be "The Strange History of a Mysterious Being and the Account of a Remarkable Journey as Communicated in Manuscript to Llewellyn Drury Who Promised to Print the Same, But Finally Evaded the Responsibility Which Was Assumed by John Uri Lloyd."[3] Both its unusual subject matter and cryptic nature caused more than its share of consternation among the reviewers of its day. If its title page alone were to be believed, it was a most amazing tale indeed, and, in fact, Cincinnati critic Charles Frederic Goss declared the book to be "one of the most striking revelations from the occult world that has been announced in modern times, if not all time."[4] Others were appreciative but not so credulous. One reviewer called it "a deeply spiritual book," and while historian-critic John Clark Ridpath concurred, he admitted that "'Etidorhpa' is a puzzle—a literary mystery."[5] The impression it left was so striking that reviewers of Lloyd's subsequent novels felt compelled to comment upon it. Social commentator and reform writer B. O. Flower praised it as a work of "vivid imagination" and for want of a better term called it a "psychical romance."[6] A few, however, were simply exasperated by its novelties. Critic for the *Dial* William Morton Payne discounted the work as "a formless and fantastic piece of fiction" whose title (Aphrodite spelled backward) "seemed typical of the unregulated sort of imagination which the book displayed."[7]

A summary of this odd tale will perhaps give some idea of its perplexing qualities. The story begins in the apartment of Llewellyn Drury in Cincinnati. There he is visited by a strange, bearded being who displays a variety of disquieting spiritlike qualities. His purpose is surprising but quite simple: to read a manuscript to his hapless host. His proposal is as follows: "I will produce it in the near future, and my design is to read it aloud to you, or to allow you to read it to me, as you may select. Further, my wish is that during the reading you shall interpose any objection or question that you deem proper. This reading will occupy many evenings, and I shall of necessity be with you often. When the reading is concluded, we will seal the package securely, and I shall leave you forever. You will then deposit the manuscript in some safe place, and let it remain for thirty years. When this period has elapsed, I wish you to publish this history to the world."[8]

Thus the plan of *Etidorhpa* is set; Drury becomes privy to a succession of fantastic communications which he, acting on behalf of the reader's incredulity, is given every opportunity to refute. To add to the mystery, Drury is told that his peculiar messenger is simply known as "I—Am—The—Man." The communique itself tells of how this once mortal man became fascinated with alchemy. "I am the man," he confesses, "who, unfortunately for my future happiness, was dissatisfied with such knowledge as could be derived from ordinary books. . . . Be that as it may, at every opportunity I covertly acquainted myself with such alchemical lore as could be obtained either by purchase or by correspondence with others whom I found to be pursuing investigations in the same direction."[9] Following this Faustian theme is his receipt of the

"Alchemistic Letter," his joining a secret society, and the rash publication of its arcane wisdom. I—Am—The—Man pays for this breach of confidence by being kidnapped, cosmetically aged, sent on a journey to the inner earth, and made an occult missionary destined to convey his experiences to a select few of each successive generation.

These amazing adventures form the bulk of the narrative and are worth explaining in some detail. After being sequestered and transported to an area near Smithland, Kentucky (obviously modeled after the Mammoth Cave region), the "adepts' brotherhood" leave him with a "singular looking being," who is eyeless with a hide the color of blue putty. It is this subterranean guide who leads him to the "Unknown Country." As they descend together, the familiar laws of nature are suspended or altered in unique ways. For example, light without either sunshine or shadows is encountered, gravity seems to vanish, and a forest with huge mushrooms is traversed. In short, all that science considers impossible or improbable seems commonplace here. The guide explains familiar laws of nature in unfamiliar ways and discusses unheard-of principles, creating, as it were, an apocryphal new world. In this land of weightlessness, unlimited energy, and telepathic powers, possibilities appear without end. But there are also dystopian elements. A macabre tale is told about a fanatical student who becomes a monomaniacal anatomist; and even more grotesque are the hallucinatory scenes after a sip of green fluid from the mushroom forest. Designed as a warning against intemperance, a series of arduous tribulations ensues. It is during this period of temptation that I—Am—The—Man meets the theomorphic Etidorhpa. "I come," she proclaims, "from beyond the empty shell of a materialistic gold and silver conception of Heaven. Go with me, and in my home you will find man's soul devotion, regardless of material surroundings."[10] Encouraged by the prospect of being with this "Soul of Love Supreme," he surmounts all trials and arrives at the brink of the "Unknown Country." At last the guide prepares to leave his charge, stating that his duty ". . . to crush, to overcome by successive lessons your obedience to your dogmatic, materialistic earth philosophy . . ." has been accomplished.[11] The finale is reached in an exuberant catharsis of emotion with yet a higher spirit escort: "Arm in arm we passed into that domain of peace and tranquility, and as I stepped onward and upward perfect rest came over my troubled spirit. All thoughts of former times vanished. The cares of life faded; misery, distress, hatred, envy, jealousy, and unholy passions, were blotted from existence. Excepting my love for dear ones still earth-bound, and the strand of sorrow that, stretching from soul to soul, linked us together, the past became a blank. I had reached the land of Etidorhpa—THE END OF EARTH."[12]

The temptation to contrast this work to the fiction of Edgar Allen Poe, Jules Verne, or even the later efforts of H. G. Wells and H. P. Lovecraft (who read *Etidorhpa* and loved it) is alluring but deceptive. Of course, most obvious antecedents are suggested specifically in Poe's *Narrative of A. Gordon Pyme* (1837) and Verne's *A Journey to the Center of the Earth* (1864). In the first, the author presents a narrative of an ostensibly "real" journey used as a literary device to propel the protagonist on his symbolic quest toward a solipsistic existence; in the second, the author uses fiction at least in part as a vehicle to speculate upon the wondrous possibilities of science as he knew it.[13] As a specific response to scientific theory and practice, however, Poe's *Eureka: A Prose Poem* (1848) offers a more appropriate comparison with *Etidorhpa* than either of these works. Even a brief perusal of the expository speculation offered in *Eureka* shows the degree to which Poe was captivated by the orthodox scientific paradigms of Kepler, Newton, and Laplace: the universe as machine. On the other hand, Lloyd was interested in promoting none of these themes, and, in fact, was diametrically opposed to the received orthodox canons of scientific praxis that supported the optimism of Poe and Verne. For this reason, comparative analyses of these authors would not reveal a great deal about Etidorhpian themes. One needs to avoid these enticing but deceptive culs-de-sac in interpreting Lloyd's first full-length novel.

Etidorhpa emerged from so-called "occult" beginnings to become a cult classic that simply refuses to consign itself to the netherworld of out-of-print fiction. But *Etidorhpa* should not be given a facile reading. The typical reader accustomed to a Victorian literature that presented extremes of either hard, empirical science or saccharine romance must have been left as puzzled as the reviewers; they simply had not seen the likes of it before. Occultists, however, were convinced of its meaning. For them the work was to be taken literally as given on the title page, and they could point to a lot of internal evidence to support their belief. How else could the facsimile reproduction of the manuscript on page 35 be explained? Then there was the seemingly legitimate map showing the location of the cavern in which the journey began on page 85. What about the cross-sectional diagram of the earth showing the exact course followed on page 331? Ignoring the fact that the author might have used all of these as literary devices to create a willing suspension of disbelief in the reader, these readers apparently needed no more convincing. The *New York World*, for example, called it ". . . in all respects the worthiest presentation of occult teachings under the attractive guise of fiction that has yet been written."[14] The nineteenth-century mystic tried to convince himself and others that *Etidorhpa* was not a literary description of an imaginary netherworld: it was an occult revelation bearing a long tradition dating from the distinguished astronomer Edmund Halley in 1692 down to Captain John Cleves Symmes's 1818 theory of concentric spheres and more recently lectures delivered by Cyrus Teed (1839–1908) on his 1869 hollow-earth vision.[15]

This latest "revelation" had been presented in a pamphlet titled *The Illumination of Koresh* and does, in fact, bear a striking resemblance to Lloyd's work.[16] Teed's epiphanic moment allegedly came when the wonders of an inner earth were unveiled to him by the "Divine Motherhood," an "experience" that, along with his emphasis upon alchemy, echoes Etidorhpian themes. Teed graduated from New York City's Eclectic Medical College in 1868, practicing medicine and "Koreshanity" through the mid-1880s at various times in towns with Lloyd family roots like Deerfield and Syracuse, New York. In short, Teed was a controversial eclectic with whom Lloyd was almost certainly familiar.

Despite their preposterous claims regarding *Etidorhpa*, the occultists have kept this book in print up to this day.[17] Thus they have historically served to both obscure and sustain the novel. Clearly Lloyd's most commercially successful work, it has been able to garner a cult following that has made it a profitable item for publishers.[18] There seems to be no end in sight. The persistence of the hollow-earth mythology, along with the emergence of the counterculture of the 1960s and early 1970s, and the rise of the New Age movement with its interest in the paranormal have created a renewed demand for the book. Leading the way was Sun Publishing, which reacquainted another generation with this strange land in 1974. Two years later an introduction was added, "The Pharmaceutical Alchemist" by Neil Wilgus. This was reproduced again in Simon and Schuster's Pocket Books version in 1978. More recently Amherst

Press included *Etidorhpa* in its inventory for 1992, and Kessinger Publishers are the latest to offer the book to the public. Lloyd's work has now been in continuous print for more than one hundred years, no small feat for *any* literary publication.

Given its longevity, *Etidorhpa* has, not surprisingly, received attention from modern critics. In addition to the brief Wilgus piece, Kenneth M. Roemer in 1976, L. Thomas Williams some seven years later, and Terence McKenna in 1991 devoted considerable attention to this book.[19] Although considered "sci-fi," *Etidorhpa* has not been ignored by the scholarly community, and their observations and assessments deserve some attention.

L. Thomas Williams views *Etidorhpa* as based upon Masonic rituals, with its main focus being a journey into the land of the dead and a portrayal of near-death experiences.[20] Kenneth Roemer, on the other hand, sees it as a partially utopian work and part of a larger aspect of the American literary landscape.[21] Perhaps most important in terms of its impact, though, is the Wilgus introduction to the Pocket Books and Sun editions. For twenty years readers have been given this gospel according to Wilgus in these readily available paperbacks. For him, the essence of this book lies in its being a description of the author's own hallucinatory experiences.[22] After a century, consensus on *Etidorhpa* remains elusive.

Still, each of these analysts has brought up important contentions that deserve to be addressed. First of all, Williams's conception of Drury's journey to the "valley of the shadow of death" is based on a brief reference in connection with the secret society's sentence passed upon I—Am—The—Man. While the idea is intriguing, it seems likely that Lloyd introduced it merely to add mystery and suspense for the reader. The fact that this "death theme" is only passingly introduced in chapter 6 and not mentioned again throughout the duration of the novel indicates that Williams has made too much of a minor literary device. Roemer's partially utopian idea has limited application, and the utopian character of Lloyd's work is easily overdrawn. The emphasis of nearly all of the utopian writers of the day was political reform. Because of fundamental philosophical differences, the novel cannot in the broadest sense of the term be considered as a part of the category of utopian reform writings found in such works as Étienne Cabet's *Voyage to Icaria*

(1840), Calvin Blanchard's *Art of Real Pleasure* (1864), or Edward Bellamy's *Looking Backward* (1888).[23] Even their approaches differed from Lloyd. Unlike these writers, whose main focus was social and political reform drawn in large part from the ideas of Robert Owen, Claude Henri de Saint-Simon, and Charles Fourier, Lloyd's focus was clearly scientific rather than sociopolitical reform. When they did examine traditional science, they were captivated *and uncritically approving.* The science fiction writers looked at science and marveled at its possibilities; the utopian writers looked at science and hoped for some realizable potentialities in furthering humankind's social and political organization: science as the formula for the perfectibility of humanity. The dystopian writers scoffed at such optimism, but they seldom offered much in the place of science other than some fanciful agrarianism. Lloyd suggested something very different from all of these groups, and thus to dwell on utopian or dystopian literature would set us upon a chase after quite unalike hares.

But this is not the only area in which Roemer is wide of the mark. He also agrees with Wilgus's argument that the work is largely a depiction of the author's hallucinatory experience with drugs.[24] Both apparently base their opinions on a note by Lloyd inserted on page 276, which reads as follows:

> If, in the course of experimentation, a chemist should strike upon a compound that in traces only would subject his mind and drive his pen to record such seemingly extravagant ideas as are found in the hallucinations herein pictured, or to frame word-sentences foreign to normal conditions, and beyond his natural ability, and yet could he not know the end of such a drug, would it not be *his duty to bury the discovery from others, to cover from mankind the existence of such a noxious fruit of the chemist's or pharmaceutist's art?* [emphasis added] To sip once or twice of such a potent liquid, and then to write lines that tell the story of its power may do no harm to an individual on his guard, but mankind in common should never possess such a penetrating essence. Introduce such an intoxicant, and start it to ferment in humanity's blood, and it may spread from soul to soul, until, before the world is advised of its possible results, the ever-in-

creasing potency will gain such headway as to destroy, or debase, our civilization, and even to exterminate mankind.

This seems to be more of an admonition against drug use than an admission of it. Furthermore, there is substantial evidence throughout Lloyd's career to suggest that he thought there was serious abuse in this regard. At one point he lamented, "The American people are now, more than ever before, terribly afflicted with new self-harmful and *habit-form-ing drugs*."[25] Lloyd was a man familiar with the power of mind-altering substances, one not likely to have experimented with dangerous concoctions.

Nevertheless, the insistence on Lloyd's personal experimentation with psychotropic substances has been carried even further by Terence McKenna in his book *The Archaic Revival* (1991).[26] Calling Wilgus's short introductory essay "scholarly and informative," McKenna insists, "There is ample evidence, both circumstantial and *prima facie*, that Lloyd had experienced intoxication by psilocybin."[27] His "evidence" consists of a very strained and self-serving extrapolation from a caption to an illustration in *Etidorhpa*: "Monstrous cubical crystals,"[28] in which McKenna finds "STRO CUB" embedded. He claims Lloyd hid the identity of his intoxicant in this caption and that it refers to *Stropharia cubensis*, one of the hallucinogenic psilocybin mushrooms. Although this fungus was not named until F. S. Earle (1856–1929) did so in 1906, McKenna suggests that the Lloyd brothers might have known about Earle's research and the name he intended to apply eleven years later. Based on this extremely weak conjecture and without researching this assertion in any depth, he concludes that "John Uri Lloyd, nineteenth-century savant, pharmacist, occultist, and author, had discovered the consciousness-expanding properties of psilocybin mushrooms, experienced them, and decided to suppress his discovery."[29]

McKenna's astounding "discovery" warrants some response. As for the caption, McKenna disingenuously implies that Lloyd's "monstrous cubical crystals" are the crystals of psilocybin formed from subjecting the crude material to boiling water at 220–228°; in fact, however, Lloyd makes it very clear exactly what this substance is: salt. The context of this illustration was to introduce some of Lloyd's ideas on the transference of salt solutions by capillary action, ideas that were duly noted and investigated by chemists Ostwald and Erbring.[30] In short, the illustration and caption so important to McKenna's line of reasoning has absolutely nothing to do with mushrooms—or even botany for that matter. The Earle connection is equally flimsy. There simply is no indication in any of the extant John Uri Lloyd correspondence that they knew one another. Curtis, the mycologist brother, knew Earle, but the only remaining correspondence between the two consists of two 1899 letters discussing general issues of taxonomic nomenclature.[31] The tone of both documents suggest a formal, businesslike relationship, not one in which intimate details of impending scientific discoveries would be shared. Throughout all of C. G. Lloyd's *Mycological Notes*, published from 1898 to 1925, Earle is mentioned only twice, and neither reference is to his *Stropharia cubensis*. McKenna's argument is simply unsubstantiated by any primary evidence.

Rather than this convoluted and somewhat fantastic thesis based on a "hidden" message and special privy knowledge of nomenclature from a mycologist one Lloyd brother barely knew, it is more likely that both John Uri and C. G. Lloyd were very much aware of the general psychotropic properties of many fungi; indeed, the mushroom scenes were probably written in on that basis. The puffball (*Lycoperdon* spp.), for example, was one of Curtis's special interests, and its narcotic effects were widely known in the nineteenth century.[32] Keenly interested in ethnobotany, the Lloyds certainly knew of the uses of a variety of mushrooms and other fungi for their mind-altering effects by shamans in indigenous cultures. They unquestionably knew of M. C. Cooke's early treatise on psychotropics published in 1860, *The Seven Sisters of Sleep*, which among other plants discusses the hallucinogenic mushroom *Amanita muscaria*.[33] It is even possible that they knew of the general effects of *Stropharia cubensis* (reclassed with the genus *Psilocybe* by Singer and Smith in 1958) and its use by the Aztecs as *teonanácatl*. Despite the fact that this knowledge was generally lost to Western science in the modern era until its "rediscovery" in the 1930s, more than a dozen early references to this plant can be found dating from the seventeenth century.[34] Those like the Lloyds with a penchant for obscure and ancient tomes might easily have been familiar with *teonanácatl*.

In light of the problematic nature of all previous interpretations, one is left searching for a theme that speaks comprehensively for its author's purpose. Here Lloyd himself provides the key. In a brief but definitive statement dictated in 1905, he sets forth the purpose of *Etidorhpa*. The author had apparently decided that the ten-year mystery should end and that a signed and witnessed document detailing not only his motivation but also the influences bearing upon the work would suffice to quash the orgy of speculation.[35] It failed. Left unpublished and unread, it has gathered dust on the shelves of his library for ninety years. Only Laurel Black has cited this important primary resource; but since hers was a study of the textual changes to the book itself and not a thematic analysis, it was never fully utilized to inform the narrative itself.[36]

Thus, it is best to let the author (in light of his "Statement") begin by indicating what his book is *not* about. First of all, Lloyd's only revelation to the mystic is that this is fiction not fact. The material for the mysterious alchemistic letter was taken from *Lives of Alchemistical Philosophers* by Arthur Edward Waite, published in 1888.[37] Lloyd then states that "the reference . . . to a manuscript left in the author's hands, is altogether a fiction." Concerning the hallucinatory scenes over which so much has been made, Lloyd rather nonchalantly indicates that he "threw in" those chapters as an afterthought. Treated as an insignificant aside and nearly left out altogether, this portion of the story has no other purpose than to demonstrate the power of chemical substances over the mind and the dangers of intemperance. These dangers were well known to a pharmaceutical manufacturer who had devoted himself to drug reform in the United States. There simply is no clear support for the theory of any personal drug abuse. Such a notion is sustained only through interpolation and conjecture based on fragmentary evidence taken out of context in a work of fiction.

The proffered critiques are clearly left wanting. Had Lloyd stopped here, the reader would remain uninformed as to his motives in producing such an odd work; but there is more. He reveals that the book was an imaginative outgrowth of his ongoing laboratory experiments and developed into an indictment against a scientific practice that had become dogma. "Authority ruled with an iron hand," he complains, "and the man who presumed to even question aloud, was likely to be crucified. In these directions I was confronted constantly with the fact that science as I found it, could not explain phenomena that came before me in my thought and work, and hence it will be seen that throughout *Etidorhpa* there are questionings and criticisms that are based upon an incredulity and even antagonism against those who at that time claimed that which they did not know, was either not worth knowing, or was not."[38] Thus stands the thesis of the work.

Unlike the social and political reform writers who presented their ideas in utopian fiction, Lloyd's target was science—scientism to be exact. He was adamantly opposed to the nineteenth-century positivism of Auguste Comte, Herbert Spencer, Ernst Mach, and others who reduced all reality to sensory perception and quantification. In its place Lloyd looked for a more satisfying replacement (vis-à-vis his eerie, apocryphal speculations) and suggested a new metascience, stripped of all positivistic materialism, that was more open to alternative paradigms. Herein lies the essence of *Etidorhpa*. Analysts may say what they will about the speculative possibilities of Lloyd's novel, but the undeniable fact is that the author himself wrote the book in protest of what he viewed as the hubris of scientific practice during the late nineteenth century.

It has been said that Lloyd's *Etidorhpa* "lies light years away from his scientific reports."[39] This is only partly true. While the book has little if anything in common with his better work in chemistry and pharmacy, it *is* akin to some of his unregulated speculative pieces as well as his polemics on any number of scientific topics. The weaknesses of Lloyd's novel read like the weaknesses of his own eclecticism as he ruminates on any number of aspects of science, not giving any real evidence of himself having any paradigmatic moorings. His speculations have a somnambulistic aspect as he bumps along from topic to topic, suggesting a concept, tantalizing the reader with its implications, and then dropping the matter altogether. Lloyd started out attempting to produce a thinly disguised treatise on the philosophy of science; what it ended up being was an overly ambitious project whose pretentious design ultimately failed to fulfill its intended purpose. Not only is Lloyd's writing stilted and his organization cumbersome, but the ideas expressed in *Etidorhpa* give evidence of an amateurish appreciation of the subjects he attempts to treat: theoretical physics, cosmology, the historiography of science, intellectual history, and philosophy. Had cultish New Agers and literary historians ignored the work, less attention could have been given to a book of such inferior quality; alas, however, *Etidorhpa* refuses to die.

Etidorhpa was Lloyd's first and last exercise in writing speculative fantasy. But his literary pen had far from run dry. Lloyd's next excursion into fiction consisted of a novella titled *The Right Side of the Car.* Published in 1897, it was written to defray the expenses of erecting a monument to his departed friend and mentor, John King.[40] Interestingly, Lloyd's trip to Tacoma, Washington, to attend the annual National Eclectic Medical Association formed the basis for this story. Eager to utilize the majesty and beauty of this region in a novel, Lloyd created a sentimental Victorian romance about a dying girl's return to her beloved home in Tacoma. This book represents a turn away from Lloyd's earlier *Etidorhpian* themes toward the local color genre that would characterize the remainder of his literary efforts.

This was a precursor to his Stringtown series, a group of six novels written from 1900 to 1934.[41] Totaling 1,775 pages, they seek to depict social life and manners in northern Kentucky around the Civil War period. The stories themselves are highly circumscribed geographically and represent an attempt to portray the people of Lloyd's youth in Boone and adjacent counties through their customs and local patois. Thus, *Stringtown on the Pike* contains all the major elements typical of local color fiction so popular during the late nineteenth century. "Theoretically," writes Grant C. Knight, "the local color story should be an objective narrative making use of facts of geography, climate, speech, and mores, but actually it often exaggerates the peculiarities with which it deals in order to entertain its readers."[42]

And entertain it did. The local color movement became almost a national obsession in the years following the Civil War and continued on into the first decade of the twentieth century. Almost every region seemed to spawn its representative author, but the South was an especially receptive field for this genre that relished delineating peoples on the brink of vast, permanent change. Merrill Maguire Skaggs has noted that certain locales are indicative of southern stereotypes: the Georgia cracker as humorous rustic, the Virginia gentry's romantic nobleman and his gentry-imitating blacks, the moody but proud Carolina tarheel, and, of course, the self-reliant Tennessee mountaineer.[43] "Kentucky," he curiously adds, "trying to have it both ways by mentioning both colonels and hillbillies, so obscures her state signals as to remain a literally borderline dark and bloody ground."

In offering a variety of characters in their works, however, the Kentucky local colorists were not obscuring their state signals but rather were signaling to outsiders something quite important about themselves and their state. If these authors could populate their works with characters as diverse as goateed gentlemen in white linen suits and barefooted country rubes, it is in large part because, as Thomas D. Clark has noted, "Kentucky has almost as many faces as there are sectional divisions of the state."[44] More than miles separate the Appalachian mountain folk from the Bluegrass elite, and each is quite different from Kentuckians of the Pennyroyal, Jackson Purchase, Ohio Valley, and Knob regions. These are the germinal catalysts that produced what can only be described as a dazzling array of local colorists in this so-called dark and bloody ground.

It should come as no surprise, then, that a man reared in a state rich in these elements should turn to a literary style particularly suited to its exploration. The years 1853 to 1863 was the period in which Lloyd as a youngster gathered the raw material for his novels. Determined by more than just place, however, Lloyd's stylistic choices were influenced in no small part by time. His birth in 1849 made him but one of a veritable bumper crop of local color writers throughout the nation also born that same year. There was Sarah Orne Jewett, whose prolific pen would give us an interesting tour of New England; Ruth McEnery Stuart's Louisiana stories; Thomas Allibon Janvier's regionally disparate tales from the Southwest and Mexico to some lesser-known haunts in New York City; Sherwood Bonner's portrayal of life in the Deep South; and closer to home, in Lexington, Kentucky, that giant of the genre, James Lane Allen. The coincidence is worthy of notice, because it places Lloyd's own work within an extremely fertile field. By the time Lloyd the pharmaceutical chemist and manufacturer became Lloyd the litterateur, local color was already writ large upon America's literary landscape.

The best way to assess Lloyd's Stringtown novels is through the stylistic conventions adopted by most local colorists. A listing of these chief attributes would include the following: a desire to observe, record, and come to grips with a variety of impending changes in their particular regions; the persistent, often excessive, use of dialect; an interest in superstition and the supernatural; a compulsion to base their writings on fact, which often results in some self-conscious intrusions into their story lines; and except for violence, a conspicuous reticence about sexuality and other themes that might be considered unseemly.[45]

The starting point, of course, is *Stringtown on the Pike*. In many ways this novel becomes the cornerstone of the entire series since many of the major characters reappear later, and even those that do not are often alluded to, as if the reader were familiar with them. In this sense *Stringtown*, while not prescriptive reading, is quite helpful in following Lloyd's other tales. The story itself covers a period from the 1860s through an unspecified time following the Civil War. Centered on Florence, Kentucky, which Lloyd changed to Stringtown because it "sounded too Italian,"[46] the novel begins with Cupe and Dinah. The peculiar interpretations of ethics and virtuous behavior by these two highly superstitious blacks play a major role in the action and development of the story. *Stringtown on the Pike* involves a sequence of subplots and a main plot concerning Sammy Drew's efforts to win the heart of Susie despite the amorous overtures of Red Head, a new arrival from eastern Kentucky. The climax is reached when the mountain boy is falsely arrested for allegedly poisoning his uncle with strychnine. Expert testimony is elicited from Sammy Drew, now a professor of chemistry from the University on the Hill, to prove the prosecution's theory. Enter Judge Elford, who attempts to spare the young chemist from alienation in his home town by asking him not to testify.

The appeal is ignored, however, and Drew's misapplied and misinterpreted forensics are used to get a conviction. In the end, though, it is a family feud rather than the commonwealth that administers the death sentence. When Red Head's rival appears in Stringtown and learns that he is about to be robbed of the "honor" due the two fighting families, the courtroom turns into mayhem as guns supplant the gallows in sealing the mountaineer's fate. The story concludes when Susie confronts Sammy Drew with the error in his test: namely, that the goldenseal root (*Hydrastis canadensis*) taken in the uncle's morning tonic produced a false positive for strychnine and the death was probably due to natural causes. Lloyd had noted the "remarkable correspondence" between the actions of strychnine and hydrastis in his scientific research,[47] and this example shows how he enjoyed incorporating his knowledge of chemistry (especially toxins) into his novels. Utterly devastated, the chemist Drew takes his takes his own life with "too dangerous a drug to be made known through science to the public,"[48] while Susie goes off to live in a Kentucky convent.

In stripping *Stringtown* to its bare essentials, a number of curious subplots have been left out. There is the intensely violent and macabre scene between a southern fire-eater (aptly named Colonel Luridson) and a person from the North, as well as the strange death of Susie's recalcitrant father, forced to take the "ordeal bean" (i.e., calabar bean), among others.

Whatever modern criticisms may be leveled against the work, Lloyd's contemporaries enjoyed the novel. William Henry Venable, the renowned literary historian who had read the story in manuscript and became something of a literary mentor to the scientist turned novelist, wrote excitedly to Lloyd, "Everybody seems to be reading 'Stringtown,' high and low, rich and poor—men, women, and children. How does it feel to be a successful author?"[49] Mention has already been made of *Stringtown*'s tremendous financial success and the ensuing windfall to the Lloyd Library, but there were those unable or unwilling to spend the $1.50 for a copy of their own. For the unfortunates who rushed to the Cincinnati Public Library to get *Stringtown*, all most could do was sign the waiting list for the 141 copies already checked out.[50]

Having created something of a sensation, *Stringtown* drew the attention of critics and even some moviemakers. Perhaps because of its obvious conformity to a style so popular in its day, it was greeted largely with praise. "Altogether," hailed B. O. Flower in the *Arena*, "we regard this book as one of the most notable works of fiction that have appeared in recent years."[51] Less enthusiastic were William Morton Payne and Firmin Dredd, reviewers for the *Dial* and the *Bookman*, respectively, the latter calling it "a curious example of how much good and how much bad a man may put between two covers."[52] Regardless of the critics' opinions, some were convinced that *Stringtown* on the silent screen would net some box office revenues, and serious efforts were made toward that end.[53]

Of course, Lloyd did not need these proceeds to support himself and his family; his financial security was assured through his pharmaceuticals. In fact, Lloyd did not initially intend to publish *Stringtown*. Instead, he planned to leave it in its original form as a three-volume typewritten manuscript entitled "The Dead Chemist," and to deposit the work in the Lloyd Library.[54] However, the publisher of the *Editor*, a writer's journal emanating from Franklin, Ohio, persuaded Lloyd that his story had merit and should not be concealed on his library shelves.[55] Despite this private encouragement and the ensuing public appreciation, Lloyd maintained his priorities and insisted upon regarding his efforts to portray his boyhood Kentucky as little more than a leisure activity: "I went at it as a matter of recreation. When I get tired of laboratory work and desire recreation, I sit down and write a chapter or two. I find it rests my mind as well as my body; it takes me out of the rut and rests me. It is about all the exercise I need. Instead of golf I find it more profitable to my bodily health to write and that is the pleasure of it. But I am not literary. I claim to be a pharmacist and I am sticking to my profession."[56]

Indeed, the rapid succession of novels that followed *Stringtown* soon threatened to escalate into an all-consuming endeavor, so much so that Lloyd abandoned his local color activity to turn his attention more fully to matters of scientific research. But this was not until several other novels were placed before the public.

Of the next three, *Warwick of the Knobs* (1901) was far and away the best; *Red-Head* (1903) was essentially a picture book rehash of *Stringtown*; *Scroggins* (1904) was a novella poorly executed and poorly received. *Warwick*, however, in some ways presented improvements over his first Stringtown novel. When the great Kentucky bookman, John Wilson Townsend (1885–1968), sought a selection of Lloyd's fiction for his classic reference work, *Kentucky in American Letters*, it was a passage from *Warwick of the Knobs* that he chose to showcase.[57]

Warwick is the story of an intransigent predestinarian Baptist preacher from Gunpowder Creek in northern Kentucky. Set during the Civil War, it is the tale of the trials and tribulations of the Warwick family. The main plot revolves around Mary Warwick, who runs away with Lionel, a "rock hunter" from the North. A shallow and insensitive opportunist, the sophisticated student/geologist soon leaves Mary pregnant and alone. The rest of the action concerns the girl's brother, Joshua, who heads north to avenge the disgrace to the Warwick family name.

Yet in the end, Joshua spares Lionel's life, realizing that his death would only spread sorrow to another innocent family. The patriarch of the Warwick household simply cannot see the matter this way and casts his son from his home as a coward. For the preacher, ethical and moral questions are black and white, a facile reasoning that gives the story a tragic ending.

This general outline does not convey the full strength of the novel, much of which is drawn from two widely divergent sources: Lloyd's perceptive treatment of historical events and his use of comic relief. His portrayal of John Hunt Morgan's raiders and many of the sentiments in the region seems to be supported by modern scholarship.[58] Clearly, Lloyd uses Warwick as a vehicle to convey his own southern-centered attitudes when the preacher declares, "God help our unhappy land if despotic might prevail over right. God help the negro when the vindictive invader tears him from his watchful owner's care and throws him helpless on the world."[59] Although Lloyd's sympathies undoubtedly rested with the South in *Stringtown*, they are given fuller expression in this novel and become a source of interest for the historically inclined reader. Other effective features of *Warwick* are its creative descriptions of city scenes unfamiliar to the rustic characters of northern Kentucky and its well-placed use of folk humor in the narrative. Lloyd's fondness for casting Joshua in the role of the wise country fool is reminiscent of George Washington Harris's (1818–1897) Sut Lovingood character.

One thing that also helps this novel work is its less obtrusive use of dialect. It plays an important part in the book, but Lloyd's white provincialisms bear faint resemblance to the patois of Cupe and Dinah, both of whom have minor roles in *Warwick*. Nevertheless, the *Warwick* dialect is not wholly effective. Its major fault is inconsistency. Mary Warwick, for example, speaks standard English, as does her father, while Joshua speaks with a pronounced dialect, one that evinces an illiteracy hard to imagine in the home of a preacher devoted to reciting scripture.

While this work has other defects—perhaps the most glaring being lapses into stilted writing—it would be unfair to criticize it too harshly. This is by every measure a much better book than *Stringtown*, an assessment supported by modern analysts.[60]

In its day, *Warwick* received praise from many of Lloyd's prominent friends and acquaintances. "Your last striking story of 'Warwick of the

Knobs,'" wrote James Whitcomb Riley, "is most welcome, in its entirety, since serially, the better the story grows, the greater my impatience over its impediment of speech, shall I call it? . . . Congratulations, therefore, as well as the best abiding godspeeds and encores of yours fraternally."[61] An old fishing buddy, former president Grover Cleveland, also showed a keen interest in the book and engaged its author in a lengthy discussion of Joshua's actions.[62]

Despite all of this private approbation, the work as a whole received far less attention than *Stringtown*. Aside from some minor coverage in the regional newspapers, most critics ignored Lloyd's second novel. The public seemed less enthusiastic as well; the Cincinnati Public Library apparently had little trouble filling patron demand. Whether readers had had enough of Stringtown and environs, or whether they simply thought that its matching tan buckram cover bespoke a companion volume that would offer more of the same, is hard to say. What can be said, however, is that the novel clearly was written within the same stylistic framework.

As interest waned, so did Lloyd's. After releasing *Red-Head* and *Scroggins*, Lloyd left fiction for twenty-six years. True to his profession of pharmacy, Lloyd knew full well that his truly important endeavors remained in scientific inquiry, *not* literature.

In 1930, however, the spry octogenarian once again returned to fiction. This time his efforts came in the form of fictionalized biography in *Felix Moses, the Beloved Jew of Stringtown on the Pike*. This is the story of a real Jewish immigrant peddler named Felix Moses (1827–1886), who comes to Stringtown and wins the hearts of its inhabitants through his kindhearted, affable ways as he runs a circuit that covers Boone, Kenton, Campbell, Gallatin, and Grant counties:

His aim seemed to be to bring the pleasure of human fellowship and good will to homes where a visitor seldom found his way, where the cheer of his countenance lighted the day for the inmates. What was needed by them he bought in the city and delivered, asking no immediate payment. He kept no book accounts, accepting that others would deal honestly with him, as he did with them. He seemed amply repaid by the welcome he received, the pleasure his coming brought, especially to the children, who eagerly looked for a sight of "Old Mose" on the day he might be expected. He took more pains, if possible, to serve the poor than those in better circumstances. Perhaps he considered that a family living in an out-of-the-way place was his especial care.[63]

This book is interesting from several standpoints. First of all, the novel is generally quite accurate historically. In recounting Felix Moses' experiences during the Civil War, the chapter titled "Fort Donelson" gives an especially vivid and detailed depiction of its capture by Union forces on February 16, 1862. Another important feature of this work is the enlightened departure from the xenophobia commonly exhibited by Lloyd's fellow local colorists. Alice Hall Petry's in-depth study of twenty-nine writers of the genre indicates that this is a typical feature of local color novels.[64] Here Lloyd stands in marked distinction. Foreign *and* Jewish, Felix Moses as portrayed demonstrates that Lloyd's pen did not exude the poison of prejudice, at least not for his white brethren.

Despite this one divergence from the local color mold, the other aspects of the novel offer the standard fare: the use of dialect; the display of regional distinctiveness; an obvious desire to observe and record events, especially those concerning the war; and a continued incorporation of the supernatural that swings back to a compulsion to base the story on fact. These last two features mar what could have been a sensitive and insightful portrait of a man and his adopted region. Unfortunately, this is Lloyd's most self-conscious work. With constant intrusions into the narrative, the author delivers various postulations, explanations, and pontifications on subjects not always germane to the subject at hand. In addition, the reader is assailed with an array of excursions into the supernatural, ranging from a personified clock that acts as a historical muse to an apparition that holds the key to a mysterious communication. In fairness to Lloyd, it should be pointed out that this novel was published locally and not intended for a large readership; it was mainly a diversion to be shared with friends, family, and associates.

Given his age and the rigors of writing, one would expect this to have been Lloyd's last work. But four years later, at eighty-five, the indefatigable author was at it again. This time it was a novel titled *Our Willie: A Folklore Story of the Gunpowder Creek and Hills, Boone County,*

Kentucky. This was actually a long-shelved sequel to *Stringtown*, which was completed to fulfill the deathbed wish of his wife Emma.[65] In many ways, this adventure/romance is much more accessible to the modern reader: The dialect is less pronounced, the plot is surprisingly well executed, humor is used to advantage in telling the story, and the paranormal is kept to a minimum. Unfortunately, *Our Willie* received little, if any, critical notice. Like *Felix Moses*, it was published locally, and Lloyd himself probably intended it for a small readership. In any case, it was Lloyd's last literary effort. Having fulfilled his departed wife's wish, Lloyd would himself pass from the scene two years later.

Taken as a whole, the Stringtown series, in spite of all its flaws, deserves to be remembered. Lloyd's local color stories were acknowledged and praised by some of the best writers of the genre: namely, James Whitcomb Riley and James Lane Allen. Moreover, these novels represent the quintessence of southern regional writing. For all his scientific ingenuity, Lloyd displayed an almost slavish conformity to this literary movement. For the literary historian wanting to understand this important class of fiction, the Stringtown series becomes too representative to ignore. In addition, it has considerable value for the historian of Kentucky. "Kentucky writers were interested in local color subjects to such an extent," writes William S. Ward, "that the beginning of a substantial Kentucky literature can be said to have developed coordinate with it."[66] To ignore Lloyd's contributions is, in effect, to exclude a seven–county area of the state from literary treatment. Even beyond this are the valuable historical accounts Lloyd gives of a region rent in two by the Civil War. Usually supported by personal recollections or those of family and friends, Lloyd gives the Civil War historian a rare, albeit partisan, view of the effects this war had on an especially vulnerable locale. Lloyd also expresses (largely implicitly) his attitude toward blacks. Although Lloyd never cast his black characters as villainous, his depictions of African Americans as childlike, superstitious, and impressionable shows that he accepted the all too common racial stereotypes held by many whites. As such, these novels become a limited but interesting window to the social attitudes of Lloyd's day.

The modern reader should not be misled. Lloyd's novels are not great literature. Those who suspect that a Cooper, Hawthorne, or Poe might be lurking behind these pages will be sadly mistaken. Lloyd's fiction is characterized by extremes: Too often what should have been the vivid colors of rural life turns gaudy with heavy dialect and overstated stereotypes; too often what could have been a bright collage of characters fades into drab formality. Still, for a man who made his living in the distant world of science, his literary endeavors merit more than passing notice and respect.

On a more personal level, Lloyd's novels served to broaden his social circle. There can be little doubt that although Lloyd never ceased being a pharmacist at heart, neither did he pass up any opportunities to cultivate his literary career or form new contacts with the literary elite. His invitation to a dinner honoring Mark Twain's seventieth birthday, for example, shows that he had truly "arrived," for the photograph published in a special edition of *Harper's* places him at the table of Twain's daughter.[67]

Of Lloyd's personal associations with literary figures, none were as important or historically significant as that with James Lane Allen. There is admittedly not a large store of extant correspondence, but those letters that remain tell a great deal about the two men at the peak of their literary creativity. They tell a rather interesting personal story not generally recognized by literary historians.[68]

Written from 1895 through 1901, these letters reflect the interaction of two men very much in their literary prime. But Allen was at this time a real powerhouse in American literature. Indeed, by 1900 Allen's reputation in American fiction was already established. While Lloyd was posting sales of 50,000 for his *Stringtown*, Allen was enjoying sales of 130,000 for his novel *The Reign of Law* published that same year. His novella, *A Kentucky Cardinal* (1894), was highly successful and, in the words of his biographer Grant C. Knight, "sounded his name on both sides of the Atlantic."[69]

The initial correspondence dated May 20, 1895, therefore, shows an interesting juxtaposition of careers. Born just eight months apart, both loved Kentucky and both dealt with Kentucky themes from firsthand knowledge. Allen was already a well-known figure and by his forties was staking everything on his literary fortunes; Lloyd, on the other hand, was an established man of science who had done little more in the field of literature than write one rather odd and eccentric piece of fantastic fiction. Allen's May letter suggests that Lloyd had sent him not his new novel but rather an assortment of scientific works, many of which were undoubtedly Lloyd's own books such as his *Chemistry of Medicines* and his *Drugs and Medicines of North America.*

Allen's expression of gratitude indicating "great personal interest" in this scientific material was more than just pro forma courtesy. Allen was very interested in what he called the "new science" heralded by Darwin's evolutionary theories, and although Lloyd would have little to say on the topic of Darwinism, the impression left by Allen's letter is that of a man steeped in the humanities seeking to draw and learn from the experience of a more scientifically trained mind. Just five years later, Allen would publish his novel *The Reign of Law,* in which he examined the implications of evolution, which he viewed as key to the future of reasoned inquiry. Allen may have had experience in the writing of fiction, but it appears that he was aware of his own limitations and quite interested in learning from a prize-winning scientist about the current state of knowledge in chemistry and the biological sciences.

This brings up perhaps the most important feature of this body of correspondence: It sheds light on Allen's character and the kind of relations he had with his colleagues. James Lane Allen has been portrayed as a stiff, distant Victorian figure, quick to take offense and seldom (if ever) warming up to anyone. The correspondence between Lloyd and Allen, however, depicts a different man. Grant C. Knight states that "Allen found himself believing that Kentucky men of letters were either pretentious amateurs or men of talent who in one way or another fell short of the mark of gentleman."[70] That assessment does not seem borne out in any of the Lloyd-Allen correspondence. On the contrary, there is every indication that Allen regarded Lloyd's work with respect and considered Lloyd a gentleman of no small attainments. "I must congratulate you in general upon the fresh activity of the past few years which have opened up for you so much happiness and the power of giving so much to others,"[71] wrote Allen. If Allen, in fact, did regard all Kentucky authors as rank amateurs or pretentious hacks, it is surely not evident in his dealings with Lloyd.

Allen's biographer goes on to insist that the famous Kentucky local colorist was essentially imperious. "At bottom aristocratic," writes Knight, "he held himself mentally and physically aloof from the crowd, and the grand manner, which Ellen Glasgow was to observe harden into a pattern upon him, was settling upon his shoulders."[72] Even earlier in his career, Allen is depicted as a man who had haughtily withdrawn from his colleagues.[73] But Allen's correspondence to Lloyd shows a collegial association, a sharing of thoughts and ideas. "I shall give myself the pleasure of coming to see you before long," wrote Allen, "and then I shall look further into your interesting correspondence and be ready, I hope, to talk with you about your book."[74]

Is this the same Allen writing to Lloyd? If Allen had been quick to take offense or disdain other authors, Lloyd would have been a good candidate. Lloyd was, after all, new to the literary scene and regarded his own work as that of an amateur. Considerably more experienced and successful, Allen could have simply ignored Lloyd as beneath his attentions, or worse, viewed him as a threat. Had Allen been so inclined, a certain amount of defensiveness on his part would not have been inexplicable, and especially so by the date of his last letter in 1901.

Although Allen's work was far and away better known than Lloyd's *Stringtown*, the dean of Bluegrass literature had already incurred the ire of many religious groups, not the least of which was the Catholic press. The source of these difficulties went back several years to the publication of his short story "The White Cowl" in the September 1888 issue of *Century Magazine* and "Sister Dolorosa" in that same publication in 1890. Both stories deal with themes of secular love and the Church, topics *not* appreciated by Catholic readers. Catholics had by 1900 already attacked Allen's handling of religious themes, and so when Lloyd had his heroine retire to the safety and solitude of a convent in his *Stringtown* novel, Catholic reviewers quickly noticed the distinct difference between the two Kentucky authors. "Prof. Lloyd is not a Catholic," observed the *Catholic Telegraph* in its November 1900 issue, "but he is a gentleman of too much honor and culture to exhibit bigotry or bad taste, as Mr. Allen and some others have done."[75] Yet Allen's association with Lloyd, even as late as September of 1901, shows no mean spirit, no condescension, no sense of feeling threatened.

It would be too much to redefine the character of James Lane Allen on the basis of his relationship with Lloyd, but the extant correspondence between the two clearly shows a man of some magnanimity who harbored no small respect for a comparative fledgling regional author. These letters also indicate a growing friendship, one that sparked personal visits that undoubtedly proved intellectually stimulating for both men as they discussed one another's work. If, in fact, Allen was the aloof, arrogant, thin-skinned man described in Knight's biography, it must be concluded that his relationship with John Uri Lloyd was atypical. The bond of respect that both men had for one another must have eluded Allen in his other personal associations, if Knight's assessment is correct. The details of the Lloyd–Allen relationship can be glimpsed only in their letters, these remaining fragments of a friendship that lasted at least during the apex of their respective literary careers. These letters, however, point to more extensive contacts, the greater portion of which may have been set down in correspondence kept and ultimately lost with John Uri Lloyd's personal effects.

Social relationships were always extremely important to Lloyd, and the diversity of his acquaintances and friendships are a measure of the man's versatility and his significance among contemporaries. Lloyd was no loner. He was a master at cultivating alliances with those who could help his career, whether literary or professional. This should not imply that Lloyd's social relations were necessarily superficial or that he viewed them merely as means to ends, but that he obviously used personal contacts well and to advantage in his career. Friends, family, and associates must be a part of any assessment of his life.

9

The Best of Times, the Worst of Times: Friends, Foes, and Family

𝒮𝓇 From the very beginning, John Uri Lloyd had the ability to cultivate important and powerful friends. As mentioned in the earlier chapters, extant correspondence with leading figures like John King, John Milton Scudder, Roberts Bartholow, C. Lewis Diehl, Albert Ebert, John M. Maisch, Edward R. Squibb, and Charles Rice shows that by his early thirties Lloyd had established correspondence and in some cases collegial relationships with some of medicine and pharmacy's best and brightest. By the late 1880s and early 1890s, Lloyd's correspondence files read like a who's who of American pharmacy and medicine; after his literary career was launched, major novelists such as Bram Stoker, James Whitcomb Riley, and James Lane Allen enlarged the list. In later years, Lloyd's prominence in a variety of fields gave him access to political figures like former president Grover Cleveland and commissioner of the Internal Revenue Service under William McKinley, George W. Wilson.

Among his more intimate professional friends, Lloyd always maintained private discussions on whatever issues were before him, conversations that motivated much of his public discourse. Thus, an examination of a few of his private relationships tells much about the public man. Moreover, these professional associations were quite consuming of his time and energies, and they could affect his family relationships. Following the death of his sixty-one-year-old father, Nelson Marvin Lloyd, on March 22, 1882, John Uri's adopted sister, Emma (now Emma Lloyd Nead of Kansas City), expressed some revealing concerns about her recently widowed mother to brother Curtis:

Mother writes me that you are now boarding over in the city [Cincinnati]. You will not think me meddlesome if I write first how I feel about your leaving [Crittenden, Kentucky]. I do not wonder at your wanting a change but it seems to me if you could have stayed with Mother through the summer, it would have been better and maybe in the fall she will come and stay with us through the winter. I think from her letters she creeps off to her room, and is alone a great deal. If you were there she would not feel so desolate. She has not said this—it is only my thoughts. You know how John's time is all appropriated, he never has a moment to bestow on Mother, and I fear Mother yearns for attention and love from us all more now than before Father's death, for then she had him to turn to with all her worryings.[1]

Curtis apparently did not heed the advice and in fact followed through with his plans to board with his older brothers in Cincinnati. Mother Sophia survived this immediate crisis and lived to the age of eighty-three. In fairness to John Lloyd, it should be pointed out that in later years he *did* make time for mother, taking her into his home in the stylish Cincinnati suburb of Norwood, where she lived out the remainder of her life. Nevertheless, whatever else may be said of Lloyd's priorities, the comment made by sister Emma reveals a man engrossed with professional affairs.

In going through all the extant John Uri Lloyd materials, there is a sense that Lloyd took great care of his wife and children without being especially intimate with his family. There are pictures of his children but they are comparatively few, and the meager supply of letters to his children suggest a relationship of stiff formality and reserve; even his grown son John Thomas always referred to "Father" with rather distant respect. If the modern reader fails to see the warmth and emotionally supportive figure expected of today's father figure in John Uri Lloyd, it is largely because such roles were foreign in the Victorian age. It is unfair to demand of Lloyd behavior commensurate with modern expectations. In those days, the responsibilities of caring for and nurturing the children fell upon the mother, while as historian Thomas J. Schlereth points out, "a majority of Midwestern fathers saw themselves primarily as reliable providers."[2] The Lloyd household typified this familiar Victorian pattern.

But Lloyd kept family matters and his professional life very separate. The essence of Lloyd—the thing that made him "tick"—was not his family but his collegial relationships. Of those associations, none were more intimate or sustained than his friendship with the eminent pharmacist Charles Rice.

Rice is one of the most mysterious characters in the history of American pharmacy. Born on October 4, 1841, in Munich, Germany, as Charles Reis, he anglicized his name to Rice upon arriving in America. Rice was a well educated, multilingual, scholarly man, but details concerning his life in Europe and his education are sketchy. Lloyd insisted Rice had told him privately that he had been "a general roustabout" on a sloop of war named the *Jamestown*, although Rice's official version was that he had served as the ship's "Surgeon's Steward." What is definitely known of Rice is that he arrived in Bellevue Hospital in New York City quite ill. Annoyed by the inactivity of his convalescence, Rice asked for some duties at the facility to pass the time. John Frey, superintendent of the General Drug Department, gave him the job of bottle washer. Rice performed his duties so well that Frey promoted him to the apothecary, and by the time of Frey's death Rice had advanced to the position of chemist in the General Drug Department. Soon he found himself both superintendent of the Drug Department at Bellevue Hospital and chemist of the Department of Public Charities and Correction of New York City.

It was a meteoric rise, but Rice had shown ambition and ability despite his hazy past. Furthermore, John Frey recognized in Rice a man of tremendous talent, and as trustee of the College of Pharmacy of the City of New York, Frey found Rice a position at the school. At this important school, he was soon noticed by other pharmaceutical luminaries such as Joseph P. Remington and Edward R. Squibb. The rest of Rice's story is well known. His role in the American Pharmaceutical Association, his chairmanship of three *USP* revision committees, and his leadership in establishing the *National Formulary* have earned him a permanent place among America's pharmaceutical giants.[3]

In this context the Lloyd-Rice friendship takes on greater importance. Theirs was not merely an idle acquaintance, nor was it a simple mutual admiration society. Rather, it must be understood that Lloyd and Rice were both leading figures in their field who frequently helped one another out on a variety of technical pharmaceutical problems. This was a powerful alliance. Their correspondence goes back to an 1878 letter concerning the processing of glycerin. The subjects of their letters soon expanded to cover a wide range of topics. The real bond between the two, already discussed earlier, was forged when Lloyd agreed to assist in Rice's important revision of the 1880 *USP*; but this was just the beginning of a long and enduring association.

Lloyd often sought the help of Rice. When Lloyd and John King wanted to quote from the *USP* in their *American Eclectic Dispensatory* but were denied permission by publisher Lippincott, Lloyd appealed to Rice as chair of the Committee of Revision.[4] Rice was flabbergasted by the refusal. "I have always understood that *anybody* has the right to quote *anything* out of the U.S.P.," Rice told Lloyd, "in fact, to quote the whole of it for purposes of illustration or comment; but the only thing he can not do is print the book *and prefix the title, The U.S. Pharmacopeia*. This title is really the only copyright."[5] Rice, well aware that John Maisch and Alfred Stillé were using the *USP* in their *National Dispensatory*, told Lloyd to query them, and concluded his letter to Lloyd with "I am really curious to learn what Prof. Maisch's answer will be, that is, how he and Stillé managed to obtain the necessary permission."[6] In the meantime, Rice would ask Squibb's advice. Squibb suggested that King and Lloyd simply ignore Lippincott, agreeing with Rice that "you would have been justified in using the whole or any part of the text of the U.S.P., *without asking permission*, for your particular purposes."[7] Lloyd's difficulties did little to endear Rice to the Philadelphia publishing house of Lippincott. In fact, an 1882 letter from Rice to Robert Amory, head of the copyright subcommittee, suggested his preference for the printing contract to go to a New York publisher.[8] This was perceived by some as exerting undue influence over the printing and copyright process, and it caused enough of an uproar in APhA ranks to prompt a motion of expunging all circulars from the Subcommittee on Copyright, a motion that was ultimately tabled. Nevertheless, the point had been made. By April of 1881, Rice wrote to John King that while the *USP* would indeed be copyrighted, "it will be expressly understood that every author will be entitled to quote from the work, either in abstract, or in the very language of the work itself. . . . Your question can therefore be specifically answered to this effect, that you will be at liberty to quote from the U.S. Pharm. whenever you wish to do so, for the purpose of adding a commentary."[9]

This example shows the lengths to which Rice would go in pursuit of what he felt was necessary justice for his friend. Lloyd understood this, and it served to deepen their mutual trust. When Lloyd's father was reported quite ill in the Ozark Mountains, for example, it was Rice he turned to for advice.[10] Most of their correspondence was of a more scientific nature. Scores of letters chronicle Rice's requests for information on various plant drugs or laboratory processes. When they were not discussing one of these topics, Lloyd and Rice would query each other about their other mutual interest in books. In fact, Rice inscribed and gave to Lloyd an original copy of Johann David Schöpf's 1787 *Materia Medica Americana*, which immediately became Lloyd's most prized possession and the rarest book in his library.[11] It is clear that both men had the highest regard for one another. Rice even gave Lloyd a standing invitation to publish any of his researches in the *American Druggist*, on which he served as associate editor.[12]

As with all close friends, politics were inevitably discussed. In November of 1884, the hotly contested presidential campaign between Democrat Grover Cleveland and Republican James G. Blaine sparked considerable comment from the two pharmacists. Apparently, Lloyd had written to Rice in favor of his personal friend Cleveland, suggesting that he reconsider his Republican faith. Rice, never one to give his opinions very freely, provides a rare and rather extended view of his political views in his reply:

> As to your letter, I must at once disabuse your mind of the idea that I am a Blainite. I have always held with the Democratic party so far as state and local politics go. In *national politics*, however, I have heretofore voted for Republican Presidents, and generally also for . . . [Republican] Congressmen (unless they were objectionable to me otherwise) for the simple reason that I did not consider the time as having arrived when the country could stand a change in *financial* policy. . . . I myself and thou-

sands of others of my way of thinking, would probably have voted for [Chester A.] Arthur or [George Franklin] Edmunds, but to vote for Blaine—no! thank you! This was too much! Therefore I was so much the more pleased when I could make up my mind to vote for Cleveland, whom I already had voted for Governor. And Cleveland will be our next President— providence permitting—there is no earthly chance to cheat him out of it! There you have my political profession in a nut-shell and I shake you mentally by the hand and exclaim: Three cheers for Cleveland and reform![13]

Rice's politics are not surprising for a professional man of science living in comfortable circumstances in the East. Blaine's connections with the corrupt railroad interests had dirtied his reputation and permitted Cleveland, who as governor had always been careful to distance himself from the political machinery of New York's Tammany Hall, to run on a clean government platform and make it believable. Historian Richard Hofstadter underscores Rice's disillusionment with Blaine's tired message: "Here was the 'Plumed Knight' of the Republican Party! A reputation built upon eulogies of the high protective tariff, which he believed to be the real source of American prosperity, on waving the bloody shirt over the conquered South, on twisting the British lion's tail for the benefit of his Irish and Anglophilic following, and on dubious and unsuccessful schemes for promoting imperialism in South America had to be protected, as though it were the most precious thing in the world, at the cost of the most desperate lies, desperately advertised."[14]

Men like Rice and Lloyd wanted efficient, businesslike government, not pork barrel legislation, rampant nepotism, and new refinements to the time-honored spoils system. Blaine symbolized every one of these all too common features of Gilded Age politics. Cleveland, on the other hand, was a fiscal conservative who opposed "free silver" and was even regarded by fellow party members years later as a Democrat who acted like a conservative Republican.[15] No wonder that men like Rice and Lloyd readily considered Cleveland their man in the White House. South-loving, Confederate-defending Lloyd must have been doubly pleased when Cleveland appointed the Mississippi jurist Lucius Lamar

(1825–1893) as secretary of the interior and the former Confederate congressman from Tennessee Augustus H. Garland (1832–1899) as his attorney general.

At one in politics, equally devoted to advancing the pharmaceutical sciences and the profession, both bibliophiles, Rice and Lloyd continued a close relationship until Rice's death on May 13, 1901. Just one month before, Rice wrote his last letter to Lloyd. Again it was an acknowledgment of Lloyd's agreement to help the *USP* Committee of Revision. "I knew you would respond to our request," wrote Rice, "and I thank you again most heartily for your assistance. . . ."[16] So closed a lifetime of gratitude from the Bellevue Hospital pharmacist.

Lloyd's professional relations were not always so intimate or even cordial. An interesting example is the Hydrastis controversy. *Hydrastis canadensis*, commonly called goldenseal, is a native North American plant with a long history of therapeutic use. It was a recognized "officinal" of the 1860 *USP* and appeared in all but the first edition of George B. Wood and Franklin Bache's *USD*.[17] They noted in 1880 that the eclectics used the "impure muriate of berberina" as "hydrastin, in the dose of from three to five grains."[18] They further pointed out that "while all admit to its tonic properties, it is considered by different practitioners as aperient, alterative in its influence upon the mucous membranes, cholagogue, deobstruent in reference to the glands generally, diuretic, antiseptic, & c."[19] In other words, hydrastis was used variously as a laxative, a healing agent in damaged mucosa, a catalyst to bile excretion, a decongestant, and a host of other uses. But the use of hydrastis preparations was not without complications. Overuse and abuse of goldenseal could produce ulcerations when used topically, a side effect noted by E. M. Hale as early as 1864.[20] Besides this, goldenseal was known—virtually distinguished—by its bright yellow color and very bitter taste. Wood and Bache further cautioned that "a more precise investigation into its physiological and therapeutic properties is necessary before we can venture to decide upon its place among medicines."[21]

John Lloyd and his brother Curtis attempted such an investigation and published those findings in their ambitious quarterly *Drugs and Medicines of North America* from October of 1884 through June of 1885.[22] This study was *and remains* one of the most comprehensive treatments of goldenseal in print. In their treatment of this plant, they noted that the resinoid obtained from hydrastis (called hydras*tin*) was "clearly distinct" and inferior to the alkaloid of hydrastis (hydras*tine*).[23] Further commenting on the various properties of hydrochlorate of berberine, the chief chemical constituent of barberry or goldenseal, they pronounced their preference for sulphate of hydrastine. "Owing to the fact that this substance can be purified without the application of heat," wrote the Lloyds, "and that it readily forms a soluble di-berberine sulphate by the action of dilute alkalies, from which other salts are easily prepared, we prefer to make this sulphate, and from it produce the various combinations."[24] The reaction of many eclectic physicians was swift. Typical was Dr. Albert Sayler of New Palestine, Ohio: "'Drugs and Medicines of North America' has exhaustively shown, to our surprise, that the resinoid Berberine (Hydras*tin*) is not a good topical agent for mucous tissues. But instead thereof, the alkaloid (Hydras*tine*) of the Hydrastis is the active property of the plant. Pray tell us," asked Sayler, "at earliest opportunity, in the Journal, what we shall do with our three dollar ounce bottles of Berberine?"[25]

Lloyd's answer was soon to come: Replace them with bottles of Lloyd's Hydrastis at $1.25 per pint. As early as January of 1886, Lloyd was advertising his "colorless" Hydrastis in the pages of the *Eclectic Medical Journal*. Touted as possessing "all the virtues of Hydrastis exclusive of the bitterness and coloring matter," Lloyd further insisted that his product was completely "non-irritating" and that it was perfectly safe to use "internally, externally, or as an injection." In light of Hale's warnings as well as Wood and Bache's caution in the *USD* that hydrastis was "bitter and somewhat acrid in saline combination," this was no small claim.[26] By February Lloyd had taken a full page of the journal's advertising section to showcase his "Authorities on Hydrastis." Here he quoted Dr. Roberts Bartholow on the superior qualities of hydrastine and E. M. Hale on his Hydrastis as "a preparation which will doubtless supersede all others." The capstone to this was Lloyd's almost prideful boast of secrecy: "Until Prof. Lloyd's process is made public, substances produced by the usual pharmaceutical methods will be different from [and by implication inferior to] Lloyd's Hydrastis." The ad concluded that "the highest medical authorities now use and recommend Lloyd's Hydrastis." These were sweeping claims for a product so new. In addition, Lloyd sent out a variety of circulars, fliers, and pamphlets to practitioners across the country, with similar professional testimonials and hyperbolic praise.[27]

The reaction of Lloyd's colleague's was predictable. Even Rice, his staunch ally and friend, questioned the wisdom of such ads and subjected Lloyd's promotional literature to some telling criticisms. "To my great surprise," wrote Rice, "several physicians of my acquaintance to whom I showed the sample [of Lloyd's Hydrastis], and who happened to look over the circulars accompanying it, at once made unfavorable criticisms regarding it, owing no doubt to some unfortunate and unwise passages in your circulars. . . . Had any other man in Cincinnati, but yourself, put out such circulars, they would have paid no attention to them, but they expressed strong surprise that *you* have done this. . . . Of course I did what I could to justify you or explain your action; but I was really powerless," pleaded Rice, "for I am *sure* you have overshot the mark. Dear friend, consider this matter well."[28]

Lloyd should have known better, especially in a pharmaceutical milieu charged with concerns for "ethical drugs" over the increasing hucksterism associated with the proprietary nostrums out on the open market. Moreover, Rice correctly pointed out that Lloyd's refusal to make his formula public caused his Hydrastis to appear on par with the spurious "secret remedies" foisted upon a gullible public. The fact that Lloyd Brothers' products were sold *only* to physicians makes Lloyd's reticence about full disclosure of this product all the more unreasonable; why not share this contribution with the scientific community? Rice's alarm was undoubtedly due to the fact that his friend's product secrecy violated a very fundamental tenet of medical ethics.[29] From Rice's standpoint, however, it was more than a matter of friendship. If Lloyd continued this form of crass salesmanship, his associations with the *USP* and the other counsels that Rice regularly relied upon could become so tainted by these patent medicine-like methods that all future collaboration with the Cincinnati pharmacist could become anathema.

Following this letter nothing happened. Then, nearly two years later, Joseph P. Remington, one of America's most powerful men in the field, exploded in anger. "I have received a communication and some circulars and pamphlets in which you are engaged in pushing the claims of your proprietary remedy, Lloyd's Hydrastis in this city and hereabouts," fumed Remington. "I very much regret to see that you are taking this method of improving your position financially, because I believe that it will very seriously injure your reputation amongst pharmacists and it certainly cannot add to the dignity of the position just now held by you as president of the American Pharmaceutical Association."[30] Remington continued the letter by nearly recanting his recent vote for Lloyd as president of the association and then (in a thinly veiled threat) told the Cincinnati pharmacist to note the constitution of the APhA, specifically pointing to article 1, sections 5 and 7.

Remington was correct in being concerned, although the specifics of his charges did not entirely apply to Lloyd's Hydrastis. While it *was* true that the preparation was *not* sold to the public but rather to pharmacists and physicians, the secrecy of the formula and the claims made for the product gave it many of the essential characteristics of a proprietary nostrum.[31] The sections of the APhA constitution referenced by Remington related to the duty of members to "suppress empiricism" and sell medicines only "to regularly educated Druggists and Apothecaries." The other section was more general and concerned the obligation of members to "maintain a standard of professional honesty equal to the amount of our professional knowledge," with the goal of the greatest good to the public.[32] Remington admitted to Lloyd that "it would be difficult to fasten upon you a charge which would infallibly convict you," but he clearly felt the spirit of the APhA constitution had been violated. Remington asked of Lloyd, "In what respect is Lloyd's Hydrastis different from Pond's Extract, or Jayne's Expectorant [two well-known nostrums then on the market]."[33] Lloyd's answer could have been simple: They are *not* sold to the general public. But such a reply still failed to address Remington's real concerns. "Now the unprofessional conduct that you are accused of," Remington added, "is that you seek to convey the impression that all other preparations are worthless, that unless the magic name of Lloyd is attached to Hydrastis that the preparation is inferior if not harmful; you have not published the full working formula, nor do you intend."

Lloyd's reply was weak and rather vague. The Cincinnati manufacturer suggested that Remington did not know the whole story and again (which was typical of him when challenged on an issue) played the martyr's part, suggesting that he had "made more sacrifices" than any other member of the APhA.[34] He did, however, promise to "excise . . . such sentences as you object to."

To understand what followed a seemingly unrelated incident needs to be examined. It so happened that Remington had just published a short article in the *American Journal of Pharmacy* suggesting that the APhA respond positively to Dr. E. Cutter's recommendation in the *Journal of the American Medical Association* that a section of pharmacy be established in the AMA. Remington saw the offer as "an excellent opportunity" for the AMA and the APhA to sweep aside "all little differences."[35] Now there was no recommendation here for an actual merger, *only a section* within the AMA. In fact, Remington suggested that the AMA could participate in APhA meetings under the section of "Medicine in its relation to Pharmacy."

Lloyd fumed over Remington's article. Lloyd raved to Albert Ebert, "Please note the paper by Prof. Remington in last Am. J. Pharm. I have every confidence in Prof. Remington's integrity, but if the move therein suggested is accepted by the A.P.A., *I will be ruled out.*" Lloyd continued, "I do not propose to become the tail to a kite, the string of which is held by a hand in the mists. I do not fear the name irregular, and, I say just wait until we give up our individuality and accept a master in the shape of the ethical and talented (?) men who run the *Am. Med. Assoc.*, and I will at once become exclusively *irregular.* I will have none of it."[36] Lloyd continued on for five more pages, warning of "any affiliation that absorbs us into the mass of this organization" and complaining, in an obvious reference to Remington, about "too much Philadelphia deference to physicians."

Now, on the face of it this was clearly an overreaction. It is true that Lloyd's affiliation with the eclectics would not have endeared him to members of the AMA, but neither would he have been "ruled out." It is also true that there was never any love lost between the AMA and the eclectics, but the proposal of mutual sections within the AMA and the APhA did not imply even the slightest reciprocal discretionary powers over the respective organizations. If Lloyd *or any other sectarian* were to be "ruled out" from the APhA, it would have to come *from* the APhA. As for Lloyd's comment about "any affiliation which absorbs us," moving from sections representing two groups to total amalgamation into one was quite a leap.

Ebert must have wondered what had gotten into Lloyd. In the context of Remington's earlier attack on Lloyd's Hydrastis, however, this letter makes more sense. Lloyd was being uncharacteristically Machiavellian here, creating a red herring to divert attentions away from his Hydrastis difficulties. His decision to write to Ebert rather than to his old and intimate friend Rice was no accident—Rice knew too much about this whole Hydrastis affair. Although Lloyd was careful to insist upon the confidentiality of his communication to Ebert, he had planted within this powerful longtime member of the APhA the ostensible motivations for a defensible exit strategy from this professional body should Remington make further threats against him. In other words, if it appeared as though Remington was not going to let this Hydrastis matter drop, Lloyd could bring up Remington's proposed connection between the APhA and the AMA as an unconscionable combination, leave in apparent disgust, and avoid even trying to defend his professional conduct within the APhA. Lloyd had already told Ebert that in his opinion the APhA had no constitution because it did not permit members to "protect themselves against their enemies."[37]

When things did not seem to move forward, however, Lloyd then alleged that some spurious circulars had been distributed without his knowledge. A postal inquiry failed to turn up an offending party, but George Lorenz of the post office summed it up best by writing back to Lloyd, "As the circular is an ad for 'Lloyd's Hydrastis' and no benefit could accrue to any one else, it would seem perfectly plausible that some one in the employ of Lloyd Bros., the proprietors of the article, would mail the circulars in question."[38] But now the whole question of authenticity and personal liability was introduced into the Hydrastis controversy. Which circulars represented Lloyd's own work? Which circulars were the productions of some overzealous employee writing and printing materials unbeknownst to the owners?

In retrospect, it seems unlikely that Lloyd was ignorant of a promotional circular being distributed in his name, and it is even more difficult to imagine anyone else printing such materials since the clear beneficiary would have been Lloyd Brothers. What seems most probable is that Lloyd saw an opportunity to plead ignorance about advertisements that were hardly defensible otherwise. Lloyd's ostensible consternation and inquiry over the ads smacks of a man retracing his steps and looking for an avenue of retreat from the field of controversy.

It seemed to work, for there is no more about Lloyd's Hydrastis after September of 1888, and extant correspondence between all parties (Lloyd, Remington, Rice, and Ebert) would indicate that all was forgotten. The product continued to be sold, however, *without* the grandiose claims. Lloyd never did reveal his manufacturing process for Hydrastis, but he also never repeated this mistake again. When Lloyd's reagent was announced, it was openly stated that "scientific data will be freely offered by both Professor Lloyd himself and by Eli Lilly & Company."[39]

If Lloyd did not take the most judicious course in the production and promotion of his goldenseal preparation, it should be pointed out that his indiscretion did not occur in a vacuum. This was an extremely rough-and-tumble, no-holds-barred business environment. He was surely not the only one ever to incur the wrath of his colleagues over the marketing of his products. One of the most outstanding examples was Frederick Stearns (1831–1907), who was formally expelled from the APhA in 1869 for marketing "a nostrum called 'sweet quinine' which contained no quinine and [was] therefore a fraudulent imposture."[40] Part of the problem was the laissez-faire business milieu of the era. One leading historian of the industry has pointed out that "market battles" and "particularly fierce" competition between manufacturers caused companies to rely "increasingly on novelties . . . to open new markets and bolster their image as scientifically advanced producers."[41] In Lloyd's case, additional blame rests not only with the temper of the times but with the product in question. *Hydrastis canadensis* continues to be plagued with controversy today. Lloyd made some bold claims about the value and safety of his product, but so do many in the field of phytomedicine today. Varro Tyler of Purdue University, one of the leading pharmacognosists in America today, insists that the near-toxic doses of goldenseal necessary to exert any discernible action in the human body make its safety "too uncertain to be therapeutically useful."[42] Yet others disagree, calling it "one of the most important native American medicinal plants."[43]

In summing up the whole Hydrastis controversy, it must be pointed out that Lloyd's actions reflected the competitive spirit of his age. The rebukes he received came in no small measure from the fact that he had always exhibited exemplary conduct and consummate discretion in marketing his products in the past. That he had one transgression should not mark Lloyd as dishonest nor as unscrupulous but merely fallible and human. Lloyd gave too much of himself and contributed too much of his expertise in other areas for this one incident to taint him in any lasting way.

One of those contributions rested in his work with the U.S. government during the Spanish-American War. On April 25, 1898, Congress, in response to a number of issues surrounding Cuban independence and jingoistic demands to flex American muscle abroad, declared war on Spain. In an effort to gain revenue for the mobilization effort, Congress passed a war tax on certain items on June 13, 1898. The key provision under schedule B of that act involved a tax on "medicinal proprietary articles and preparations."[44] The original suggestion of the government was to set the tax at 4 percent of the retail price, the same as it had been during the Civil War. After considerable lobbying by the Proprietary Association of America, a compromise was struck at 2.5 percent.[45] What followed was a long list of items to be considered under the provisions of this act, which included not just proprietary medicines but also cosmetics and related drugstore products. Not surprisingly, some of the headings from this formidable list were general and rather vague; the problem remained of which products were to be liable under this tax as *proprietary* products and which were not. In inexperienced hands, the problem of applying this tax to specific pharmaceutical items was impossible, and in fact, the IRS staff had already done a fair amount of bungling in the matter. George W. Wilson, the commissioner of the Internal Revenue Service under President McKinley, turned to John Uri Lloyd. Admitting that "none of us people here know anything about the medicine business,"[46] Wilson knew that Lloyd Brothers products were not sold to the general public and were therefore exempt from the provisions of schedule B, thus avoiding any conflict of interest on Lloyd's part.

Nevertheless, Lloyd wisely agreed to assist in this process in secrecy; had manufacturers found out about Lloyd's work, undue pressure and requests for favors could have easily ensued. Lloyd reviewed the situation and found it such a mess that he told Wilson he would take the whole problem back to Cincinnati where he would work through it from scratch. This he did, but in the meantime, Wilson and the attorney general repealed all previous rulings and awaited Lloyd's recommendations. Working in conjunction with the attorney general, Lloyd compiled lists of items subject to taxation (all those not listed were exempt). "Under these circumstances," writes Lloyd, "the manufacturer himself would know, without bothering you [Wilson and the IRS], whether or not he should put the tax upon this or that preparation."[47] Although the war had been over since December of 1898, the so-called stamp tax on proprietary medicines hung on. Not surprisingly, the Proprietary Association of America complained about the government's inconsistent application of the law and urged its repeal.[48] But Lloyd had worked long and hard on the problem of differentiating the products then on the market into proprietary and nonproprietary categories. The government's satisfaction with Lloyd's work permitted the assistant attorney general, James E. Boyd, to make a very clear distinction of proprietary items within the vast body of pharmaceuticals of the day. "It might make the distinction still more plain to say that the class of medicines which, in my opinion, are taxable under the law," Boyd announced, "are such as . . . [those] which go to the consumer in the unbroken packages in which they are put up by the proprietor, manufacturer, or compounder, with name, disease, and directions for use without the intervention of a prescription of a physician or pharmacist."[49] No matter how clearly enunciated, the Proprietary Association took the predictable stand that the tax should be removed posthaste. Finally, schedule B covering this class of taxable items was eventually repealed on February 28, 1901.

Lloyd's work with the U.S. government in secrecy was in some measure an extension of his more public associations with politicos under Grover Cleveland. Lloyd was a regular member of Cleveland's Bass Island fishing retreat party, which included Leroy Brooks, Admiral Robley Evans, and former secretary of the treasury Charles Foster. Lloyd's association was an informal one, but it was unmistakable and duly noted in the press.[50] This made Lloyd's name a known entity among government officials; yet because of his role as a man of science, he could escape the label of being a mere Democratic partisan. Thus, no one under McKinley's Republican administration hesitated to rely upon Lloyd with the war tax issue. Lloyd's national connections spilled over in local politics as well. He was a member of the grand jury that was part of a general municipal campaign to clean up government following the collapse of George B. Cox's political machine in Cincinnati. This, plus his association with Cleveland's "good government" image, caused a committee of reform-minded Cincinnatians to offer Lloyd the mayoralty in the name of the Democratic party. Lloyd had no political aspirations and quickly declined, but his pharmaceutical colleagues took note of this unusual offer to one of their own.[51]

As the first decade of the twentieth century progressed, Lloyd continued to pursue his professional activities, not the least of which included his role of providing a degree of leadership to eclecticism. To show how far Lloyd had come from his defensive posture in 1888 in the Hydrastis affair, he was acting as champion of the new National Pure Food and Drugs Act passed by Congress on June 30, 1906, which prohibited the manufacture, sale, or transportation of adulterated or misbranded food and drug products. Additionally, the act transformed the *USP* and *NF* "officials" from de facto status (long recognized by the pharmaceutical and medical communities) to de jure status by declaring any preparation adulterated if "it differs from the standard of strength, quality, or purity, as determined by the test laid down in the United States Pharmacopeia or National Formulary official at the time of investigation."[52] It was not quite that simple, however, for a "variation clause" gave manufacturers a loophole if a named *USP* or *NF* drug *different* from current standards stated plainly on the label the *actual* strength, quality, or purity of the contents. It also permitted unofficial drugs (i.e., those not named in the *USP* or *NF*) to conform to their own standard. The act was far from perfect, but it was the most important piece of legislation to date on the regulation of food and medicine in this country.

Lloyd's part in what has been commonly called the Pure Food and Drug Act of 1906 was that of liaison between the pharmaceutical and medical professions at large and eclectic practitioners. Lloyd spelled out his unqualified support of the new act in the *Eclectic Medical Gleaner.*[53] Lloyd insisted that everyone—pharmacist *and* physician alike—be held to the provisions of the law. "It is necessary to the law's vitality," he insisted, "that no one be exempted. Should physicians be excluded from its penalties, the law concerning imposters would fail. Many pharmacists would also be exempted, for numbers of these are physicians."[54] Lloyd added, "The greatest harm done the people . . . is accomplished by persons sailing under the name *physician*, or by adventurers, who employ physicians in order to get their business legalized."

It is interesting to note that Lloyd indicated that the law itself would not cause sweeping alterations in the eclectics' preparations. He found only two internal and two external medicines affected by the provisions of the Pure Food and Drug Act, which required the manufacturer to list on the label both the presence and amount of opiates and other substances deemed dangerous. The two products intended for internal use included diaphoretic powder, which contained nineteen grains of opium to the ounce, and sudorific tincture, which contained ten grains of opium to the ounce. Long "official" in the eclectics' *King's Dispensatory*, these preparations could conform to their own standards of strength and purity but needed merely to add clearly on the label the grains of opium contained therein. The two external remedies, opthalmic balsam, which contained one grain of morphine to the ounce, and mild zinc ointment, which had two grains of morphine per ounce, were likewise subject to the same regulations. "Not an Eclectic remedy carries a secret narcotic or heart depressant," concluded Lloyd, "nor does one contain a coal-tar synthetic. Not an Eclectic remedy has been changed in composition in order to conform to the National Law, nor is it necessary that one be so changed."[55] Addressing the National Eclectic Medical Association at its thirty-eighth annual meeting in Kansas City in June of 1908, Lloyd declared, "This law is designed simply to make men who are not honest, honest in the statements they make concerning their goods, and not to disturb any one who is fair in business. That is the object of the law. We stand today just as we stood then. We are no more concerned about this Pure Food and Drug Law than before it went on the books," Lloyd concluded, "for there is no mis-statement regarding any remedy you gentlemen prescribe."[56] It would be difficult to verify Lloyd's statement with regard to each item in its materia medica, but if true it would stand in marked distinction to the vast body of pharmaceuticals then on the market. According to a 1911 survey, for example, nine thousand samples of six *USP* drugs found roughly 45 percent in noncompliance with current standards. One year later a larger sample uncovered 31 percent in noncompliance with standards.[57]

Besides championing the Pure Food and Drug Act cause in 1906, Lloyd also left for an extended trip abroad. On February 17 Lloyd left with his wife and two daughters by steamer for Naples. This trip was taken under the auspices of the U.S. Department of Agriculture and the Smithsonian Institution "for the purposes of carrying on scientific botanical investigations."[58] Eclectic physicians followed Lloyd on his trip through his series of "Foreign Letters" that appeared in the *Eclectic Medical Journal* from May through July. From Italy, to Turkey, to the Middle East, Lloyd took notes and observed the cultivation, transportation, and processing of crude drug products from their indigenous locales. Lloyd returned from his travels on July 20; he later reported on his overseas investigations to the APhA and wrote a number of articles drawn from that experience.[59]

Remembering Lloyd's *Etidorhpa* and his speculative challenge to mainstream scientific paradigms, one is inclined to believe that this eclectic—this scientific dissenter—might be sympathetic to non-Western ideas and perhaps might even view the magic and mysticism of the native peoples with a nonjudgmental eye. Yet this trip would produce no "Tao of pharmacy."[60] What it *did* produce was much of the foundational research for his book-length study, *Origin and History of All the Pharmacopeial Vegetable Drugs*. Interestingly, Lloyd railed against what he saw in his excursions beyond the American pale. Far from the sophisticated citadels of learning, Lloyd found conditions deplorable. "God help the people who depend on such medication and such medicines as this Old World and this Oriental World possess," he wrote in his last "Foreign Letter."[61] "Never until now," he added, "have I been in a position to know what the American physician possesses, over the world at large, in the line of therapeutical advantages. Like an oasis in a desert came before my eyes, in one of these cities, a welcome sign led me to stop, to read, to turn and read again: '*The American Pharmaceutical Specialties of Parke, Davis & Company sold here.*'" In the end, Lloyd showed himself to be, if not a *regular* in the healing arts, a thoroughly *orthodox* scientist. What Lloyd failed to notice (or perhaps deliberately ignored), however, was the fact that the universities of Europe, especially in Germany, were revolutionizing education and research in medicine. The dramatic changes being heralded by the new biologicals and synthetics were changing the foundations of modern pharmacy. But Lloyd had *arrived*, had indeed already made his contributions to the field.

Lloyd gave poignant testimony to this fact at the Hotel Pennsylvania in New York City on April 19, 1920. In his Remington address before the assembled throng of APhA members, he exhorted: "Keep the Home Fires Burning."[62] Here it was that Lloyd's peers bestowed the highest award attainable for an American pharmacist. He was only the second so honored, and it was a fitting acknowledgment of his life of service in the field of pharmacy. Lloyd told the audience of his debts to W. J. M. Gordon and George Eger, who laid the foundation for the "country-bred boy of sixty years ago." He then eulogized the medal's namesake, Joseph P. Remington. In thinking over his remarks, Lloyd must have harked back to his difficult days in 1888. But now, more than thirty years later, those professional wounds had long since healed. Now Lloyd was being given a medal bearing the name of the man who had once threatened to oust him from the very organization that was granting its greatest distinction. Remington surely represented for Lloyd the best of times, the worst of times.

But the home fires that Lloyd alluded to in his speech were casting their light in different directions. Lloyd made repeated references in his address to "ideals of the past, and service to the present"—where was the future? The world had changed since Lloyd first entered pharmacy, and it was continuing to change. By 1920 Lloyd was the last remaining leader in eclecticism. Lloyd might hope for the home fires of his therapeutic faith in vegetable materia medica to be rekindled by the next generation, but by the 1920s the fires of eclecticism had already ceased to cast their light on modern medicine; theirs was a fire that smoldered with the remembrance of past achievement and former accomplishment. Nevertheless, this luminary was not quite ready to be extinguished. Some contributions were yet remaining in the pen of the last great eclectic.

10

The Last Great Eclectic

By the 1920s, the recent Remington medalist had established an imposing array of contributions to pharmacy. This manufacturer, teacher, and author could easily have rested on his laurels. But Lloyd was forever restless, forever inquisitive. He was *never* idle; this was particularly true regarding unfinished business.

One such item related to investigations launched by Lloyd years before as part of his series of articles, "Precipitates in Fluid Extracts." Those award-winning studies had touched on a number of areas that Lloyd had long suspected as trailblazing. Lloyd had observed that absorbent paper immersed in an aqueous solution of lead acetate, and a variety of other mixtures similarly tested, produced distinctive separation patterns on the paper. In itself this was nothing new. Christian F. Schöbein (1799–1867) and Friedlieb Runge (1794–1867) had described this kind of capillary chromatography years before. What *was* new, however, was its application to pharmaceutical processes. Lloyd utilized these chromatographic principles and found that a "solvent can be perfectly separated from dissolved matter by what appears to be simply capillary action."[1] He further pointed out that "this dissociating force has been overlooked in many places where, perhaps, it might have been useful. It may have been an unknown factor in leading to discrepancies in delicate analytical work that involved frequent filtration."[2] This process of capillarity may be described as "a phenomenon associated with surface tension, which occurs in fine bore tubes or channels," examples of which include "elevation (or depression) of liquids in capillary tubes and the action of blotting paper and wicks."[3] Given the nature of capillarity itself, it is no wonder that Lloyd naturally came upon this activity as part of his laboratory work.

Despite the potential of using capillarity in pharmaceutical processing, Lloyd did little to pursue his investigations following 1885, the last of his "Precipitates" articles. He was, however, curious about how much work had been done in this particular field, and so with Sigmund Waldbott he launched into an exhaustive bibliographic search of the relevant literature. The labors of Lloyd and Walbott yielded 665 annotated citations. Their *References to Capillarity* remains one of the most extensive reference sources in its field.[4]

What they discovered was that Giovanni Borelli (1608–1679) demonstrated an inverse relationship between the height of a fluid rise and the internal diameter of the tube. These observations were refined by Francis Hauksbee (1666–1713) and James Jurin (1684–1750). The physics of capillarity was examined in depth by Johann Andreas von Segner (1704–1777) while at the University of Göttingen and by Ludwig Leidenfrost (1715–1795), who described the phenomenon of surface tension. Studies in capillarity were carried on in the nineteenth century by Pierre-Simon Laplace (1749–1827), who published his work on the subject in 1806, and also by Thomas Young (1773–1829) working in England. Coextensive with Lloyd's own work in capillarity was that of Hungarian scientist Roland Eötvös (1848–1919), who developed a method for precisely determining surface tension. All of Eötvös's work on capillarity was published between 1876 and 1886.[5]

Although Lloyd must have recognized that his work was new in its pharmaceutical applications, his investigations into capillarity remained unfinished until the 1920s and 1930s. He resurrected them briefly in 1917 with an article titled "Solvents in Pharmacy." Admitting that publication in this subject had ceased with his 1885 essay, Lloyd was encouraged by Wolfgang Ostwald (who, it will be remembered, reprinted Lloyd's original work in his *Kolloidchemische Beihefte* in 1916) to continue the series. Lloyd actually made few additions to his discussion of capillarity other than some marginal comments in footnote form, but he did see the significance of his contribution and its potential quite clearly. Noting "this neglected section of pharmacy," Lloyd pointed out that "little, if anything, has yet been accomplished to assist those who propose to study the comparative capillarity and connected influences and attributes of different solvents on different drugs used by pharmacists."[6] Other than this observation, however, it would be wrong to conclude that Lloyd had done more with capillarity in this essay other than reintroduce the topic to the profession.

There is little more on this topic until 1928, when the APhA noted that Ostwald had continued Lloyd's work in capillarity and *confirmed*, under controlled conditions, many of Lloyd's original observations.[7] Finally, Ostwald and Walter Haller used Lloyd's original work as the basis for a new series of studies in capillary activity in pharmacy.[8] Further elucidating Lloyd's observations on surface tension (i.e., the phenomenon that causes a departure from a flat surface where a liquid meets a solid), the German chemists presented "sixty-one photographs of menisci of the most varied origin, which completely confirm and supplement the former subjective observations [of Lloyd]."[9] In further studies, Ostwald and Haller confirmed Lloyd's description of the physical properties of glycerin, various alcohols, acetone, chloroform, acetic and sulfuric ethers, benzine and benzol, carbon disulphide, turpentine, and petrolatum as solvents for certain plant constituents; and they also substantiated Lloyd description of "pendant drops" in chemical solutions.[10] Ostwald and Hans Erbring's work took some interesting turns. Noting a curious little exercise involving the transference of salt solution through capillary action described almost playfully by Lloyd in his fictional work *Etidorhpa*, Ostwald and Erbring concluded that what Lloyd called "spontaneous" transport of liquid had some far-ranging applications:

> It is evident that if this phenomenon can be seen to rest on a safe experimental and possibly also theoretical basis, it will be of interest in many a question of physical and colloid chemistry. The senior author himself (*loc. cit.*) [John Uri Lloyd] has pointed out that such movements of liquids would affect geological and hydrological questions, e.g., as to the origin of salt lakes and subterranean water courses, thereby assuming that porous materials like sand, sandstone, etc., act in the same manner as filter paper. Then the theories of "swelling" suggest themselves. Concerning this, different authors, e.g., Procter and Wilson, J. Duclaux, D. Jordan Lloyd, J. Loeb, Northrop and Kunitz, etc., have recently considered "osmotic" forces in the movement of water

in the swelling of gels although the existence of "cell structure" or "semipermeable membrane" in swelling gels has not always been proved, nor is it even always considered probable.[11]

These researches carried Lloyd's work in physical chemistry forward. It is important to emphasize, however, that these studies undertaken by Ostwald, Haller, and Erbring were confirmations of less systematic descriptions made by Lloyd in the 1880s. As such, they truly represent the work of these German chemists and *not* the work of Lloyd. Nonetheless, they do show the value of Lloyd's keen powers of observation, and Lloyd *does* deserve credit for introducing the subject of capillarity and colloidal activity to the pharmaceutical sciences. Lloyd's contributions were fully recognized by leaders in the field of colloidal chemistry. When Jerome Alexander compiled his massive six-volume reference work, *Colloid Chemistry: Theoretical and Applied* (1926–1946), it was Lloyd who contributed a section titled "Colloids in Pharmacy."[12]

Curiously, although Lloyd's colloidal work connected with the reagent that bears has name has received wide attention in pharmaceutical circles from the very beginning, the same cannot be said for his observations in capillarity, surface tension, and other aspects of physical chemistry as it relates to pharmacy. This is probably due to how the topic evolved within the field. Colloids were not given extensive treatment in *Remington's Practice of Pharmacy*, for example, until 1936.[13] By that time, Ostwald, Haller, and Erbring had already taken Lloyd's lead and verified many of the pharmaceutical applications of this specialty. Lloyd's role in this process has been blunted by the fact that these important studies were diffused over a period of time and then carried forward by others. Nowhere were they brought together as a complete monograph. Today the topics of capillarity and colloidal chemistry as they relate to the pharmaceutical sciences are covered extensively, and Ostwald is correctly considered the leader in these fields.[14] Yet the acknowledged doyen of colloidal chemistry himself stated that "modern physical chemistry confirms and proves in a beautiful manner the observations Professor Lloyd made so many years ago."[15]

Unfortunately, other aspects of science would prove less kind to John Uri Lloyd. While Lloyd was devoting himself to the details of perfecting his phytochemical processes in extracting natural plant products for his Specific Medicines, other areas were moving forward in ways that would dramatically transform pharmacy. Advances in organic chemistry, microbiology, endocrinology, and immunology were bring- ing on a host of new synthetic and chemotherapeutic agents. The bark of *Salix* spp. (willows), for example, had long been known for its anti- pyretic and analgesic properties because of its salicin content, but Her- mann Kolbe (1818–1884) led the way in synthesized drugs when he made salicylic acid in the laboratory in 1874, making it cheaply available for the first time. By the time Ludwig Knorr (1859–1921) produced antipyrine in 1883, Germany was on the cutting edge of pharmaceutical advancement.[16] In the 1890s, Emil von Behring (1854–1917) succeeded in producing an antitoxin against diphtheria, thus heralding a new class of therapeutic serums.[17] In 1910 clinical trials showed that arsphenamine (Salvarsan), synthesized in the laboratory of Paul Ehrlich (1854–1915), was an effective antisyphilitic agent. By 1935 the synthetic Prontosil was shown to be effective against streptococcal bacteria, ushering in the so-called sulfa drugs.[18]

The reaction of the eclectics to these modern innovations was less than enthusiastic. In fact, while the pharmaceutical profession had long since come to terms with the germ theory by 1900,[19] eclectics even as late as 1905 were "poking fun at microbiology as the new religion and Pasteur as its god."[20] John King Scudder, son of Lloyd's mentor, John Milton Scudder, suggested that "a good old medicine or method is not quickly thrown over for a new and untried one."[21]

Lloyd's response was interesting. Initially at least, he seemed to fully appreciate the contributions of the German chemists and their synthet- ics. "The advent of salicylic acid, antipyrine, antifedrine, salol, etc., indi- cates that there is a future in this direction that those persons whose interests commercially are only with nature's crude productions will do well to consider," Lloyd observed. "As it is at present," he admitted, "Germany has the advantage. The patient investigations of years in the German universities is being rewarded by discoveries that may prove of greater commercial value than we can foresee. Already the world at large is sending millions of dollars to that country for such substances as sub- stitution dyes, salicylic acid, and other bodies that I have named; and I, for one, will freely concede to them a right of return."[22] Later, however, after the eclectics had sent their volleys against the germ theory and other modern concepts, Lloyd recanted. In 1908 Lloyd reduced the "patient investigations" of the Germans to "a little cloud" that arose in that country from their discovery of synthetic salicylic acid. Instead of conceding their "right of return," Lloyd now accused them of producing "untried monstrosities."[23] Lloyd continued to oppose these therapeutic "faddists" and their "intoxicated followers" in subsequent issues of the *Eclectic Medical Journal.*[24] It was unfortunate that Lloyd, so innovative himself and so intellectually acute, should follow the eclectic fold so slavishly. That Lloyd in his heart and soul knew better is evinced in his first remarks on the subject back in 1888. Lloyd's professional identity with the eclectics usually served to elevate the sectarian group above its ordinary level of mediocrity; in this case, though, the ball and chain of eclecticism's anachronisms kept Lloyd from moving forward with his profession. Indeed, while innovators like Rudolph Buchheim (1820–1879) and John J. Abel (1857–1938) were ushering in the new science of pharmacology, Lloyd was still clinging to traditional notions of an American materia medica, an empirical and didactic study that had always "ranked rather low in the pecking order of medical subjects."[25]

By the 1930s, the last great eclectic was ready to pass from the scene. He had lost his brothers in 1926 and he was turning uncharacteristically inward. Much had to do with his own health. A fungal infection in both ears from years before had left him so impaired that by 1930 he was turning down dinner engagements because of his "blunted hearing."[26] By the time his wife of fifty-two years died on November 27, 1932, Lloyd was frail and failing. He seemed to have but one unfinished earthly obligation: fulfill the deathbed request of his wife Emma and complete the last of his Stringtown novels, *Our Willie.* He accomplished this in 1934, but in its pages we see the loneliness of a man who had lingered past his three score and ten:

> Return to the village of your childhood after years have passed.
> Note the faces of the residents who have taken the places of the
> companions of your youth. Nearly all are strangers to you and
> you to them. Wait a year, more or less, and the word "nearly"
> must be erased. But the most melancholy feature of your
> thought of the past will be that strangers have taken the places
> of beloved companions—strangers who give you a sidelong

glance of curiosity as you pass along the way. Such is the course
of life, as we all must discover. This is doubly true to him who
is so unfortunate as to have outlived his generation.[27]

Lloyd did not have long to wait. After a fall in his home in Cincinnati just prior to the Christmas holidays, he went to the home of his
daughter Annie Welbourn in Van Nuys, California. At nearly eighty-
seven, Lloyd had lost his resilience. Finally, on April 9, 1936, having developed pneumonia, he quietly passed away. His body was cremated and
the ashes were sent to his beloved Florence, Kentucky, where they were
interred at Hopeful Cemetery.

The death of this last great eclectic marked the effective end of an
era. By the 1930s, eclecticism had fallen behind in the three critical areas
of modern medicine: education, professional identity, and technology.
The fact that these three areas lacked coherent paradigms throughout
most of the nineteenth century saved and indeed perpetuated eclecticism, but by the twentieth century all that had changed. Abraham
Flexner (1866–1959) had provided a standard for medical education in
advocating university-based instruction augmented by strict adherence
to scientific method and laboratory analysis; professional identity was
solidified in a large and alluringly co-optive AMA against ever-weak-
ening sectarian affiliations on both the state and national levels; and the
technology of medicine stood on a firm foundation forged by the watershed discoveries of Rudolf Virchow, Robert Koch, Louis Pasteur, and
others during the last quarter of the nineteenth century. By the 1930s,
medical science was moving rapidly on very new diagnostic and therapeutic fronts. "The eclectics in contrast drifted into a position increasingly contemptuous of change," observes historian John S. Haller, Jr.,
"truculent, slow in accepting new knowledge, and comfortable in mus-
ing about the past. Having become overly cautious in disposition and
argument, the reformers propounded a dialectic that was apologetic in
its defense of traditional medicine—a role reversal that occurred without fanfare and without critique."[28] Unable to compete in the new age
of medical education, the Eclectic Medical College was cited by the
Council on Medical Education and Hospitals of the AMA for numerous deficiencies in a letter of June 21, 1935. Finally, the AMA agreed
to credit graduates of the EMC subject to official dissolution of the

school.[29] The graduating class of the Eclectic Medical College on June 7, 1939, would be the last.[30]

With John Uri Lloyd gone and eclecticism all but vanished from the medical scene, Lloyd's manufacturing concern was surprisingly still in business. While most companies had enlarged their staffs to include a sizable cadre of scientific researchers working to develop new biologicals and chemotherapeutics, Lloyd Brothers remained essentially unchanged: a small, specialty house primarily manufacturing botanical medicines.[31] The firm of Lloyd Brothers Pharmacists, Inc. (the official company name after 1924) was sold to the New York botanical house of S. B. Penick in 1938, against the wishes of John Thomas Lloyd. In October of 1938, John Thomas made an effort to enter his father's realm as John T. Lloyd Laboratories, marketing a line of "Lloydsons" products. Penick's ensuing lawsuit forced John Thomas Lloyd to cease distribution of any "trade mark 'Lloydson' or any other colorable imitation or close simulation of plaintiffs' trade mark 'Lloyd' and 'Lloyd's.'"[32]

The S. B. Penick Company took advantage of the Lloyd name recognition for many years thereafter. But time marched on, and by mid-twentieth century the firm was a mere shell of its former self. Lloyd Brothers has been described as a firm that by 1960 "still sold 18 outmoded botanical medicines together with a few more modern drugs, mainly hematinics, laxatives and digestive aids."[33] When the German pharmaceutical company Hoechst was looking for a door into the U.S. market, it cast an interested eye on the old Cincinnati botanical house. The chief lure was the active and resourceful marketing staff of the firm, a team that was able to post a $1.8 million sales figure for Lloyd Brothers' products in 1960. That same year, Hoechst purchased Lloyd Brothers for $4 million in cash, changed the name to that of the parent firm, and moved operations into new, modernized facilities. Ultimately, the Cincinnati plant was closed down to consolidate with the main headquarters in New Jersey.

It is tempting to see the demise of Lloyd Brothers in T. S. Eliot's anticlimactic terms: "This is the way the world ends / Not with a bang but a whimper." But Lloyd's lifetime of work cannot be so summarily discounted. When the collapse of this long-standing botanical specialty house is viewed within the larger context of pharmaceutical development during the first half of the twentieth century, such an assessment stands like a gross oversimplification. There were much larger forces operating against Lloyd's phytopharmaceutical work.

Varro E. Tyler has recently pointed out that "echinacea is reasonably typical of the fate of 300 or more classic plant drugs during the years 1900–1962."[34] The chemotherapeutic drugs, the new pharmaceuticals emanating out of serological investigations, and the new class of antibiotic agents were causing a therapeutic sensation in Western medicine. "The direct antimicrobial effects of these new drugs were easily demonstrated," continues Tyler, but "such was not the case with echinacea, which functioned by an entirely different mechanism. By 1962, echinacea was as obsolete as a drug could be in the United States even though research data supporting its utility as an immunostimulant was beginning to herald its renascence in Europe." In contrast to echinacea and other natural products, however, pharmaceutical companies rushed to patent the latest laboratory innovation in antibiotics or chemotherapy.

Thus, it is too simplistic to simply dismiss Lloyd Brothers' products, or more important, Lloyd's medicinal plant research as the remnants of a bygone era. Rather, at least in part, they fell victim to a time when certain laboratory techniques provided for the patentable processes of medicines that netted manufacturers enough economic incentive to develop more of the same. Most medicinal plant products were not as amenable to patent protections. This fact combined with the eclectics' anachronistic resistance to modern medical praxis to cast virtually all botanicals as outdated. Lloyd's uncritical acceptance of eclectic objections to therapeutic innovations worked against both his firm and against phytomedicine generally.

Despite this fact, Lloyd stood in marked contrast to this sectarian group. "What immediately sets Lloyd apart from other individuals prominent in Eclectic pharmacy . . . ," notes Alex Berman, "was his conviction that chemistry had to be applied to the problems of Eclectic pharmacy."[35] Indeed, it was Lloyd's systematic approach to medicinal plant analysis that separated him from eclecticism's pervasive mediocrity and yielded lasting contributions to pharmacy in general. If Lloyd had disassociated himself from these eclectic idiosyncrasies and had used his resources to create a large research and development infrastructure devoted to phytopharmaceuticals in the same manner that other companies were applying to synthetics, the future of his medicinal plant products might have been brighter. As it was, however, Lloyd was spending inordinate energies and finances on shoring up a lost cause.[36] In any case, what should be emphasized is that Lloyd's products did *not* fail to survive necessarily because they were ineffective; some may have lacked efficacy but surely not all of them.

Lloyd passed away in a milieu that pointed away from the traditional vegetable materia medica, but much of his research remains sui generis. While investigators such as Daniel Hanbury, Friedrich Flückiger, and Alexander Tschirch certainly labored alongside Lloyd in their efforts to advance our knowledge of medicinal plants, Lloyd's writings in the field remain important to the present generation of researchers.

There is little doubt that the Western world is in the midst of what some are calling an "herbal renaissance."[37] As in the popular grassroots movement of sectarian medicine in antebellum America, consumers are turning to self-help over-the-counter herbal products as their first line of defense against illness. Retail sales of herbs in the United States at $1.5 billion speak to this popular enthusiasm for natural product therapies; in Europe the figure is as high as $6 billion.[38] As a response, phytomedicine is appearing in a proliferating number of professional symposia, workshops, and panel discussions, not to mention a growing presence in the scientific literature.

Not surprisingly, Lloyd's original examinations of various plants for medicinal use are resurfacing. Most directly is the rebirth in 1982 in Sandy, Oregon, of the Eclectic Institute, Inc., a company that is committed to reprinting some of the original eclectic literature along with disseminating current information on botanical medicine. More generally, however, Lloyd's work on a host of plants is being verified today. Most notable is the example of echinacea. Lloyd was introduced to the purple coneflower by a physician from Pawnee City, Nebraska, whom he described as "an illiterate empiricist."[39] Nevertheless, Lloyd was intrigued by the claims made for the plant and subjected it to more systematic analysis. His published findings for echinacea as a remedial agent against infections and "septic conditions" has been recognized by current pharmacognosists like Varro Tyler as an important scientific contribution.[40]

Some of Lloyd's other medicinal plant studies are being borne out in the current literature. His examination of the hawthorn plant (*Crataegus* spp.) for cardiac disorders, for example, is substantiated in the European community, especially Germany. "There are many prepared remedies," affirms Max Wichtl, "in which extracts of this drug, often combined with extracts from hawthorn leaf and flower, form an essential part. The more than 100 preparations are mainly in the group cardio-tonics, coronary remedies, antihypertonics, and arteriosclerosis remedies, geriatric remedies, and tonics."[41] Indeed, Lloyd's indications for skullcap *(Scutellaria lateriflora)*, a plant often dismissed by the medical community but which has received extensive treatment in Russia, correlate to a large extent with recent findings. Studies verifying its use to "normalize blood pressure" and as an efficacious remedy for insomnia, restlessness, and other "nervous diseases," echo Lloyd's discussion of the plant as a general "nervine" and stabilizer in "intermittent pulse and palpitation."[42]

The point is that John Uri Lloyd's work still has relevance today. The legacy of Lloyd in pharmacy is that he appreciated the contributions that laboratory analysis could make in phytomedicine and yet he adopted a broad perspective with regard to his investigations. Long before ethnobotany was established as an independent academic discipline, Lloyd was applying its principles in his work. "When a tradition exists among a people, a tribe or a section year in and year out touching on the use of some herb for a specific disease, I have always approached the subject with an open mind," admitted Lloyd. "Hardly a day passes," he added, "but we receive letters from doctors or the laity who tell us of the use of some drug in their neighborhood for some purpose—clinical evidence often apparently unbelievable, but still often proving true when proper research is conducted into it."[43] Lloyd's catholicity allowed him to roam freely among the plant kingdom without preconception or prejudice. This combined with his commitment to scientific methodology and his gifts in laboratory technique to yield significant results and make Lloyd the leading and most widely respected of the eclectics.

Yet as this narrative has shown, Lloyd's connection with this botanical sect was both a hindrance and a help. On one hand, Lloyd's association with the eclectics was the catalyst for his appreciation of and interest in America's indigenous plant materia medica, but on the other hand, Lloyd's single-minded devotion to eclecticism burdened him with an ideological baggage that forced him into a defensive position that was increasingly out of step with modern medicine. These attachments were formed early in Lloyd's career and rooted deep within his own character.

EPILOGUE

Beyond the Persona, Beneath the Mask

Yale University's Sterling Professor Emeritus of History Peter Gay has written an extremely perceptive analysis of Victorian society. The very first line of his book *The Naked Heart* announces the compelling thesis of the work: "The nineteenth century was intensely preoccupied with the self, to the point of neurosis."[1] Through countless diaries, autobiographies, histories, portraiture, and other "exercises in self-definition," Gay shows how the Victorian bourgeois—both powerful and petty—were preoccupied with introspection and confessional catharsis.

John Uri Lloyd epitomizes this characteristic of the age. Virtually all of Lloyd's writings, even his most dispassionate scientific treatises, have an autobiographical air about them, as witnessed in his frequent use of the pronoun "I." Whatever his expository prose was elucidating, Lloyd persistently reminded the audience of his intimate involvement with his subject matter. This is all well and good, but Lloyd's frequent personalizations present the historian with the same difficulties attending any work of an autobiographical nature. "An autobiography is a complex speech act," observes Gay, "often a triumph over anxiety, cajoling, apologizing, boasting, all in the name of narrating a dependable personal history. But, quite apart from other incentives for distortion, the sheer passage of time often inflicted on the autobiographer a persona that hardened into a mask."[2]

This surely happened to Lloyd, and in many ways it was deliberate. Lloyd carefully crafted a persona that depicted him in a context that verified popular notions of survival of the fittest. Rising from obscurity in the backwoods of Kentucky, Lloyd wrote a description of his rise to prominence of which Horatio Alger would have been proud.[3] The real picture was somewhat different. His humble beginnings, rustic though they were, need to be placed within the context of his comparatively well educated parents, whose modest but comfortable existence afforded young John a head start that certainly exceeded that of the average American lad. Also, Lloyd's apprenticeship, while undoubtedly arduous, was no more so than most, and his pay was comparable to that of the average apprentice of the 1860s. His entrance and rise in pharmacy was not without hardship, but he forged strong and powerful alliances early on, and his successes far outweighed his failures.

Nevertheless, Lloyd cast himself as constantly struggling against adversity, and when he allied himself with eclecticism he could augment that image with a leitmotif of persecution. In short, Lloyd enjoyed playing the role of rebel with a cause and reveled in his associations with sectarians who could easily be cast as underdogs. In an address before the Ohio State Eclectic Medical Association—a speech frequently reprinted—Lloyd repeatedly reminded his colleagues of his sacrifices for eclecticism.[4] Lloyd told his audience that "it is well known that no man has felt more severely than have I the persecution of authority that in pharmaceutical ethics (from my standpoint) once misled the majority. Authority that I honor still," he added, "and grant was looking only to the good of pharmacy, erred, I believe in its ethical teaching, and I suffered much criticism in consequence of my heterodoxy."[5] Lloyd advertised his eclecticism proudly: "I am satisfied to have my name go down in history as one who has spent his life as a member of the minority in more directions than one; and I believe that as I have shirked no responsibility, I have earned my full share of reproach, if there be any reproach, in the part that you and I have borne as workers in the eclectic section, the minority school in medicine."[6] Lloyd concluded his speech by conjuring up images of the sacrificial martyr: "Even if I stand alone I shall maintain my principles, and in the future as in the past I shall do that which I believe to be the right, regardless of any personal abuse or harsh criticism that may follow this stand."[7]

This persona was cultivated even in his private correspondence. Writing to Edward Kremers, for example, Lloyd grumbled, "I have no reason to regret having been traduced and abused in behalf of fact, but, really, I would not like my boy [John Thomas] to go through what I have passed."[8] Even in a simple thank-you note to Rufus A. Lyman, the great pharmaceutical educator from the University of Nebraska, Lloyd whined about receiving "nearly a lifetime of 'cold shoulder,' from men of learning and science."[9]

In the context of Lloyd's three Ebert Prizes, his presidency of the APhA, his collaborative work with various pharmacopeial revision committees, his teaching at the College of Pharmacy—all mainstream achievements and activities distinct from his eclectic affiliations— Lloyd's complaints seem like the worst kind of ingratitude. As for receiving the "cold shoulder" from scholars, he was offered a full-time professorship at the University of Wisconsin and refused.[10]

Lloyd was never neglected by his peers, but deep within the Kentucky-boy-made-good there was a nagging sense of inferiority. One cannot psychologize too much about why a man of Lloyd's stature should feel this way, although some of it probably stemmed from his lack of formal education. Lloyd always suggested that those with empirical knowledge knew as much if not more that those with formal schooling.[11] By 1907 Lloyd was also cautioning against the "illogical stress placed on some features of this entrance scheme" at medical schools.[12] Yet Lloyd knew full well that "education was never more necessary than now, and the trend of the science side of pharmaceutical education has been and is upward, towards greater skill and higher qualifications, and our country is being filled with young pharmacists with better general educations and more scientific endowments, but less practical experience, as a rule. . . . I admit freely," he concluded, "that the methods of college instruction are superior to those of former times and that in a general sense the courses are more exacting."[13]

But what of this man with *no college education*? It will be remembered that Lloyd found his lack of formal education a topic about which he felt the need to "absolve my parents from neglect." When faced with the well-read, multilingual Charles Rice and John Milton Scudder, or the Philadelphia College of Pharmacy alumnus Joseph P. Remington, or the German university-trained Albert Ebert, Lloyd must have felt somewhat ill at ease with these contemporaries. Sometimes in his private correspondence, Lloyd would all but admit to these feelings. He wrote to Edward Kremers, for example, that "I have smarted under the self humiliation, but, my dear Prof., circumstances prevented me from getting educationally what others more fortunate received."[14] It was typical of Lloyd merely to offer the complaint with no concrete explanation to the whys and hows of these "circumstances," but it undoubtedly bothered him. Lloyd's career reflects Alex Berman's assessment of the nineteenth-century botanico-medical movement in general: a striving for respectability.[15] This might go a long way toward explaining what would compel a man to publish and republish articles and editorials numbering up to five thousand, as if his lack of formal education could be erased by the repeated printing of his name. It helps explain the library he created and his pride in offering it to the public at large. It also sheds light on Lloyd's excursions into literature. None of this should diminish Lloyd's outstanding library nor his efforts at writing fiction, but all were surely calculated to make up for what Lloyd viewed as embarrassing educational deficits.

Nevertheless, Lloyd was at heart a pragmatic laboratory analyst whose keen powers of observation allowed him to pursue new facets of pharmaceutical processes and phenomena. He even demonstrated a talent for capturing the essence of local color fiction and became a brief but beloved literary sensation. As a teacher, he could command the respect of students and colleagues alike and was remembered fondly by graduates years later.

Lloyd was all these things, and he was a self-made scholar. This meant that he did have certain limitations. He did not, for example, have a thorough understanding of broad interdisciplinary concepts. His weak grounding in theoretical aspects of the biological and chemical sciences left some of his work to be verified by others like Ostwald. But Lloyd had practical skills that made him a hands-on scholar capable of making lasting contributions to the scientific literature. Lloyd's innate mental agility and facility for laboratory manipulations that yielded practical results outweighed his lack of formal training. Despite his achievements, Lloyd sometimes engaged in behavior that shocked other scholars. Lloyd was so concerned over professional appearances and public image, for example, that he took it upon himself to destroy key letters between himself and Charles Rice. "I went over my correspondence especially that with Dr. Rice," he told Edward Kremers, "and with a few exceptions, destroyed all the letters I had received from him that could have made an unpleasantness in any direction. Goodness knows there is enough left that an indiscreet or unfriendly historian might employ for sensational purposes."[16] This truly rattled the Wisconsin professor of pharmacy, a scholar with an acute interest in the history of his discipline. "As to any 'indiscreet or unfriendly historian' making use of such correspondence for 'sensational purposes,'" replied Kremers, "this can easily be guarded against by making certain letters unavailable until after a lapse of years. In any case, however, I think that the truth is better no matter how unpleasant than ignorance. . . . To place a man on a pedestal he does not belong, I think is just as much a crime as to make use of information that does not redound to the credit of such a man."[17] Kremers was so bothered by Lloyd's disregard for historical documentation that he brought the matter up again in a subsequent letter, arguing, "No doubt historians will sometime find information about the events which you desire to kill through silence."[18] Lloyd never got the message; he truly did not care that the destruction of his valuable correspondence could be damaging to future scholars.

Given all of Lloyd's faults, however, he still stands as a remarkable man. His development of practical pharmaceutical processes and apparatus was significant: His innovations with fuller's earth developed a pharmaceutical product marketed by Eli Lilly for forty years. His textbook *The Chemistry of Medicines* is recognized as one of the first books of its kind to emanate from an American pen. His book *Elixirs* was a precursor and catalyst for the *National Formulary*. His experiments with surface tension, paper chromatography, and adsorption/absorption were appreciated as pathfinding innovations when first examined and later verified by the leader in colloidal chemistry, Wolfgang Ostwald. And his researches into medicinal plants and crude drug products are still very pertinent to today's researches into modern phytopharmaceuticals. Perhaps most important of all is the library he bequeathed to society, at two hundred thousand volumes one of finest and most comprehensive collections in pharmacy and botany in the Western world. Scholar or not, his is an imposing array of accomplishments and contributions for anyone.

The quotation that opened this book indicated that Lloyd felt his biography should tell more than the story of his life; it should take one down many different "side studies." Indeed it has. Following Lloyd's life has shed light on the history of American pharmacy during a pivotal period of its development. It has revealed the many facets of this complex discipline in all its competitiveness, excesses, and deficiencies. Yet it has also revealed its efforts at professionalization, its attempts at product standardization and purity, its concern for ethics, its manufacturing development, and the revolution in its therapeutics following the paradigmatic transformation of modern medicine. Lloyd's life has also taken us down a brief chapter in America's literary history, a period when regional distinctions were fast disappearing and authors were racing to capture and preserve them in fiction. We have followed these trails because Lloyd himself walked down each one of them. Sometimes he strayed from the well-worn path to show a new approach; sometimes his trailblazing led to a cul-de-sac. He was, alas, human, but he was a remarkable man. His diverse interests, his versatility, and his partisan spirit all yield only one conclusion: He was in every sense of the word eclectic; indeed, he was the great American eclectic.

APPENDIXES
NOTES
BIBLIOGRAPHICAL ESSAY
INDEX

APPENDIX I

Remembering Lloyd's Specifics

Lloyd's Specific Medicines held a long and enduring place for the compounding pharmacist. There are few left who remember these specialty drugs, now long passed from the scene. While the historian is compelled to give "the big picture," which includes the context of their development and their place among competing pharmaceuticals, it must be recognized that in the final analysis the purpose of Lloyd's Specifics—indeed of *any* medicine—is to be prescribed and used. In this sense, the reminiscences of those who dispensed it can be valuable and illuminating. An example comes from the pen of Ken Klaiber, a retired Cincinnati pharmacist (Cincinnati College of Pharmacy, class of 1937) who was kind enough to share his memories of Lloyd's Specifics' place in the old neighborhood drugstore.

My memory of Lloyd's Specifics goes back to the 1930's when I was a student at old Woodward High School downtown and at the Cincinnati College of Pharmacy. My father operated a corner pharmacy near historic Grammer's Cafe in the "Over-the-Rhine" section of Cincinnati. In those days there was a drugstore at every corner. For everybody the drugstore was a short walk from home. We lived in an apartment adjacent to the pharmacy. I grew up in a drugstore.

In those days Lloyd's Specifics were important medications and occupied an important position in the prescription department. They were all liquids in square, space-saving bottles. In my memory I can clearly see those names: Aconite, Buchu [Barosoma], Cimicifuga [Macrotys], Capsicum, Digitalis, Ergot, Guaiacum, Hyoscyamus, Hydrastis, Ipecac [Ipecacuanha], Jalap, Lycopodium, Podophyllum, Stramonium, Taraxacum, Uva Ursi, Viburnum, and many others. The active ingredients of several are still in use today, including Digitalis and Hyoscyamus.

One of Lloyd's products enjoyed widespread use, not only by eclectic physicians, but throughout the medical profession. It was an ointment called Libradol [an "antiphlogistic and local analgesic"]. It was packed with sheets of parchment paper which was wrapped around skin areas where the ointment had been applied.

Pharmacists were delighted to dispense Lloyd's Specifics because they were the most profitable items in the store. Physicians would prescribe 30 to 60 drops of two or three Lloyd's Specifics and lactated pepsin in a quantity sufficient to fill a four ounce bottle. The cost to the pharmacist was just a few pennies. The prevailing price to the patient was 75¢.

A Modern Drug House

Dr. John Fearn, an EMI graduate, class of 1877, has provided posterity with an unusually detailed description of an early twentieth-century pharmaceutical manufacturing plant in his account of Lloyd Brothers' operations. Although the letter is undated, several comments by Fearn make it fairly easy to estimate the year of writing. Fearn's mention of the construction of a new library on Court Street, his reference to the "pure food law," plus his mention of William Holden as librarian make 1907 the probable date of authorship. No changes to spelling have been made in transcribing Fearn's letter, but punctuation has been modernized to lend clarity to the narrative.[1]

My father was not a physician, he was a mechanic. But he was a great nature lover, and very early he taught me the names and medical properties of many of the plants growing around my home. Small wonder then that I early found myself making herb teas, infusions, and decoctions from these plants; small wonder that this love of vegetable pharmacy should follow me to this day. That early love was fostered by the teachings of Scudder, King, and Lloyd, whom I have elsewhere designated as the *Three Johns*.

From my first introduction to Prof. J. U. Lloyd, our acquaintance has been of the pleasantest character. I knew of the firm when it was Merrell, Thorp, and Lloyd (also when it was Thorp & Lloyd). But since it has been Lloyd Bros., my dealings and experience with each member of the firm has been of the most ideal and pleasant character.

In my early experience on the Pacific coast, I could not get Specific Medicines. The wholesalers did not keep them and would not because they said there was no call for them. I said I would make a call. As at that time I had a drugstore, I sent to Lloyd Bros., got Specific Medicines, and let the Drs. know I had them. In a short time there was such a call that the wholesale houses put them in stock, and for a long time now it has been easy to get them on the coast.

In the early part of September of this year, I found myself in Cincinnati after an absence of more than 30 years. I was soon at the old stand, but what changes had taken place. For 4 days I went in and out, sometimes under the guidance of Prof. Lloyd, at other times alone asking questions of the workers. These workers without exception were most courteous to me, never seeming to tire of my questions. I was so delighted with what I saw that I determined to write a brief account of this busy and scientific hive so that many who use their drugs might have an idea of the place from whence they come.

In the large room on the corner of Court & Plum Sts. I found Mr. Ashley Lloyd in charge. I hesitate to say how long he has held down that job, for you might say he was an old man. The fact is he is not old, though I admit he is getting older. In his very pleasant circumstances & remarkably pleasant company, it looked to me as though Ashley was renewing his youth, for he sheds a genial smile that lights up the whole place.

Near him Mr. J. Bell has his desk. He is Business Manager and Buyer for the firm. He has been there many years and seems likely to grow old in their service.

Then scattered around the room are the desks of 12 or 15 young ladies. Typewriters, accountants, correspondents, and in a sheltered corner sits a young lady at the private exchange telephone desk. Wires connect that desk with every point of the establishment, and the outside world is reached by two other private wires. As you look around here, we seem to hear a voice which says Business!—Business!!—Business!!!

Next we find the city sales room, where medicines are shipped and packed to Drs. and Druggists all over the city and all over this great land. *But no Retailing*, and let me here say a good word for the packers: in an extensive experience breakages are kept to the lowest minimum.

The next story of the five-story building carries general medicines and chemicals, which are here ready for distribution. The story above this carries powdered drugs, pressed herbs in broken, also in full packages, from ten pound boxes to a cask. Next comes an entire story devoted to laboratory work, from washing bottles to finishing specialties. It also contains the poison department, where all the poisons are stored, labelled with *Red Labels*, and every care taken for their segregation and safety. On this floor is also the *Printing Department*. When labels & c. are printed, this might be thought to be an easy thing to print labels by the thousand and have done with it. But since the passage of the pure food laws, every batch of alcoholic preparations must be assayed for its alcoholic strength and the percent of Alcohol in every case must be placed on the labels, so that the printing of labels becomes a very different thing to what it was in the old days, as the percentage of Alcohol will differ in different batches.

Next we have a story for finishing & filling remedies. Here in systematic order are formed a great stock of remedies that are in constant demand and which are being sent to all parts of the country. Here we see large stone jars holding fifteen gallons each, all hermetically sealed to prevent evaporation. These are for special demands and emergencies and the filling of small lots. In a retired corner of this floor is to be found the office of the *Wizard* of the establishment, John Uri Lloyd, busy at his desk attending to correspondence and wrestling with the problems of the Laboratory, which are his especial care. On this floor is the Assaying Department under the care of a competent chemist, Miss Mary Stewart, and her assistant. Here are tested all the energetic remedies which must conform to standard strength *Alcoholic* and *Alkaloidal*. At the time of my visit they were testing a fresh batch of *Spec. Piper Meshysticum* [i.e., *Piper methysticum*, or the kava plant], and as I have long used this remedy, I was much interested.

Passing from this building to the upper floor of the large building on the corner, we are at once in the manufacturing department. Here are great percolators with a capacity of from five hundred to one thousand pounds each of crude materials; these percolators are connected with stills and condensors that to the [un]initiated seem very complicated.

Passing down to the floor below, we find this floor filled with large copper percolators connected with the condensing apparatus to bring the remedies to their prescribed strength. Here we see percolators holding not less than one hundred and fifty pounds each in sets of three, bearing the names of well-known remedies. As we look around here, we see the great need of systematic methods in running an establishment like this. In this large room a multiple filling apparatus is found. The machine works automatically. By pulling a lever, one hundred bottles are filled in five minutes.

Here is one of the largest acid proof jars in America. It was made by the *Daulton Pottery Co. of London*. It stands so high that for the convenience of the workers the floor below is cut away, thus the jar is set in the story below. In this jar is mixed Lloyd's Hydrastis, 1,500 pounds at a time in a room below specially prepared for this purpose. The entire batch is bottled in a few hours by a specially devised bottling machine, the liquid being filtered as it comes from the floor above.

Passing now to the floor, below we find the largest of pharmaceutical apparatus copper tinned inside. The percolators hold from one to two tons each; they are in sets of two each connected with a concentrating apparatus, which automatically exhausts the drug and brings the preparations to standard strength. When the percolator holding say 2,000 lbs. of Gelsemium is being extracted, the one holding the drug previously worked is being emptied and cleaned, ready for the next filling of this or any other drug. A walk here while these manipulations are going on is certainly well calculated to fill the mind with wonder.

During your visit from place to place, you cannot but be struck with the thought that every one of these employees seems to understand his business. Having completed one task, they seem to know almost by intuition what comes next, and without uncertainty everything seems to go like well arrainged clockwork. You see here the skilled hand, the educated brain, the perfection of the most complicated machinery, and everything under the control of that *Wizard* sitting at his desk in the office of the fifth story.

Having thus gone from floor to floor, all too hastily I admit for my own pleasure and profit, I went to another building on another street. Here are stables of mills and apparatus for grinding and mixing and sifting drugs and the places where I saw crude drugs piled up on boxes and barrels all carefully segregated and labelled, awaiting their turn to be made up to supply the wants of progressive physicians all over the land. Here is also the *Libradol*[2] department, one of Lloyd's latest medical creations but already so important as to demand a separate establishment systematically conducted for its elaboration.

As I have tried to recall the above facts in connection with my delightful visit to this place, certain thoughts come trooping up. First, when I think of the bulk of medicines that are being made here all the time, and that the bulk of these are used in very small doses, I ask myself the question, what becomes of it all? Of course an examination of the books of the firm would only answer the question. Remember that this firm does not make pills or other specialties of this character, their work being liquid and powdered medicines. [When] I think of that imense acid proof jar taking fifteen hundred pounds at one dose of *Hydrastis canadensis* (and this only one preparation) and then all that is being used by other firms for different purposes, I am not surprised that Hydrastis has gone up in price, so that good crude is worth ——— per lb. I remember years ago discussing this subject with "Prof. Lloyd." I told him I believed the time would come when, if it was not cultivated, the supply would be exhausted. He told me then he had been making provision against that day. On a farm, under favorable circumstances of soil and conditions, he had set out his beds of Hydrastis, and I think when the government of this great country through its agents gives attention to the perpetuation of our native medicinal plants, they are in good business.

The second thought that impressed me was the care in every department to secure as far as possible *Aseptic conditions*. The floors, the tables, the apparatus were all clean, and so far as I could see, scrupulously so, considering the nature of the work. The employees were not frowsy and dirty or slouchy, but as neat and bright as employees could be. In this connection, let me call to your attention the production of *Aqua Destillata* [distilled water] both for the firm's use and for their trade. The apparatus is of special design. The water from the still is caught in a compartment glass encased so that no impurities from the surrounding atmosphere can enter. This apparatus is silver plated inside even to the tip of the tube from which the water flows into the bottles. The water is allowed to flow into the bottles at near boiling temperature so that it is absolutely sterile, then stopperd while hot; as a further precaution, each bottle is further tested for impurities. I ask this question, could care go any further than this? It seems to me the festive germ and microbe must have a hard time at Lloyd's.

There are other features upon which I might dilate, but time forbids. But

I must just give you the benefit of one condition that impressed me greatly. That was the delightful social, kindly, cordial, and sympathetic feeling between employees and employed. I never saw anything equal to it. I have known places where just as soon as a member of the firm have in sight, a signal would be given and everyone would be on his good behavior and hard preparations would be made to be seen at their best. J. U. Lloyd seems to be the presiding genius over the whole factory, and everywhere he is received with signs of pleasure. All are at home with him, even to the youngest messenger boy. Everything that could affect the comfort of the employees seemed to be done. Was it a hot day, was it a cold day, was it a wet day, so that the young ladies did not want to go out to lunch? A boy was detailed to interview them, then go outside to get milk, bread, fruit, meat, or whatever they might wish. Filtered ice water was within the reach of all. To these little things I was witness: gas stoves were handy to make coffee or tea or to warm lunches; for those who enjoyed reading, there is already the nucleus of a small library for use during the lunch hours. As the result of all this kindness and consideration, are you surprised that their employees stay with them? Once in a while lightning strikes and a fair girl is led away by some fortunate swain to the marriage Alter, and generally speaking her career so far as pharmacy is concerned comes to a sudden stop—but the men, how they stand by. Some of them have a record of over 25 years with the firm.

Up to the time of the passing of the pure food law, a girl would have to be on the waiting list for a position for a year or more. Since then the business of the firm has been so much increased that the force in both office and laboratory have been increased. In addition to what I saw inside, I learned outside of things that could not help but make and cement the good feelings here seen. Vacations are given, on more than one occasion the sick had been cared for by the firm and nursed back to health, and some of the employees had been aided to get their own homes. Prof. Lloyd takes a very close interest not only in their skill and physical well being but also in their moral welfare, and I do not believe there is a young lady in their employ but what could go to him with any problem that she could not take to her father. I would like to thank every one of those employees from the lowest to the top floor for their courtesy to me. I have a picture gallery; I carry it with me wherever I go. That gallery supplies me with scenes and faces that look down on me by night and day in summer and in winter. While I have this gallery I am never alone, and since my return from the Queen City, I have other pictures I have hung there—scenes from the laboratory which to me are better than a theatre with the most superb settings. There is also another picture of an old friend in a new setting—he is a small man [with a] nervous temperament [and] pale face piercing through kindly eye and loving heart, and as I think of him going about among his work people, I give him a new name: *The Little Father*, otherwise J. U. Lloyd.

Perhaps I should not close this paper without a brief reference to the Lloyd Library. The Bros. Lloyd have not only worked for themselves. Theirs has not been a mere struggle for money itself, but for money that shall benefit others as well as themselves. There was no necessity for them to take their money for such an enterprise as this. But they have planed *[sic]* wiser than they knew, and this institution will keep their memory fragrant long after their bodies have gone to dust. I have for some time had a desire to see this institution. It stands on Court Street, the block just above the laboratory building. At the time I visited it, it was not a good time to form an estimate of its worth. The building is a substantial four-story building, and it was supposed it would be large enough for its purpose for many years to come, but it is already overcrowded and ground has been broken for a building on Court St. right opposite the Laboratory, where with better facilities the capacity and usefulness of the building can be more than doubled. The afternoon I was there shelves and tables where *[sic]* loaded & books were piled on the floor awaiting more commodious opportunities for their arrangement. It will help us to get some idea of the extensive character of the library if we note that in this library there are already more than five hundred pharmacopeas gathered from different parts of the world. The libraries of America as well as those of the old world have been ransacked to secure the treasures here found. Here is to be found as near as possible every book that can be found that concerns plants or plant products or the record of drugs. Captain Holden, the librarian, is in charge, who is ever ready to extend help and information to visitors. Prof. Aiken, also a Botanist, is here to lend completness to the institution. His attention is given to classifying plants and to naming botanical specimens sent for identification. To this Mecca come scholars and scientific men who find here data they can find nowhere else. Here adulterations and sophistications may be scientifically studied, as well as the therapeutic actions of drugs.

The museum of Mycology or Fungi (in same building) is more extensive than any other such institution in the world. Mr. C. G. Lloyd devotes his entire time to the study of fungi, the most difficult of all plants, and is now the world's authority on the subject. He spends much time in the Kew Museum, London, and the museums of Paris and Berlin, where his talents are recognized as they are in America his homeland. And so the talents of these Bros., each in his own sphere, are continually shedding lustre on our cause, which is the cause of scientific and progressive medicine.

Ostwald's Note

The following is a complete English translation of Wolfgang Ostwald's introduction to his German-language edition of John Uri Lloyd's work on percolation, precipitates, capillarity, and colloids, which appeared in the *Kolloidchemische Beihefte*.[1] The author gratefully acknowledges the assistance of Mary Jo Fasold and Dr. Thomas H. Leech for the translation.

Editor's Note

The following treatise is the translation of a series of studies, the first of which was published 37 years ago and which appeared in the Proceedings of the American Pharmaceutical Society from 1879 to 1885. Prof. J. U. Lloyd, in response to the special request of the publisher, agreed to a second publication of at least the greater part of these investigations, which were originally presented in the form of a public lecture. After revising the studies and arranging for their republication in a limited edition, Prof. Lloyd left the choice of the parts to be translated to the publisher.

Actually, it is not historical interest which prompted the publisher to ask Prof. Lloyd for a new edition of these studies. Likewise, the fact that these studies were familiar to only a small circle, because of the limited circulation of the medium of their publication, was not a deciding factor. Rather, it is the publisher's opinion that in these studies, in which "something new in regard to everyday phenomena" (Ch. Darwin) is found and discussed with truly exemplary insight and with penetrating acumen, a direct connection to our contemporary questions of the day appears self-evident in many places. For example, recently the question of the origin and the effects of turbidity in pharmaceutical tinctures has been heatedly discussed. As far as the publisher is aware (and he is interested in these phenomena for other reasons and has therefore reviewed the relevant literature), nowhere, not even in the handbooks and pharmacopoeia is to be found anything which even approximates the complete, detailed, copious discussion of the responsible factors than is to be found in the present treatise of J. U. Lloyd. The remarks of this researcher on this subject, as well as his remarks concerning the theory of percolation, the interesting experiments on the influence of the percolator's dimensions on the output etc., are composed in such a way that large parts should be incorporated completely into the text-books about the manufacture of pharmaceutical preparations, in which very little on this topic is actually to be found. Furthermore, the phenomenon of the Liesegang Rings[2] and in general the appearances of periodic, spatial disconti-nuities accompanying spatial processes that are in theory continuous, such as chemical reactions, precipitations, crystallizations, congelations etc., belong to the list of currently debated topics in colloidal chemistry. In these studies, J. U. Lloyd describes perhaps the simplest and therefore perhaps the most important attempt of this kind in terms of theory, yet to be published. It suffices to add sugar syrup to a test tube half filled with water (whereby the syrup sinks to the bottom and after a short time, produces a solution that becomes increasingly diluted toward the top of the test tube) and to heat this system from the side in order to produce after some time, strikingly clear layers of sugar solution with varying degrees of refraction. Of course, this is not even the simplest un-published attempt in this field, of which the publisher is aware. Prof. J. U. Lloyd demonstrated to the publisher in his laboratory in Cincinnati, a test tube, in which distilled water revealed three to four distinct layers which originated in the test tube as a result of continuous heating of the top and cooling of the bottom. There is no question that a more exact experimental and theoretical analysis of the causes of the origin of such layers in progressively decreasing fields of force is also of utmost significance to the more complicated case of the Liesegang Rings. To a certain extent, the present treatise contains the analysis of these phenomena which appear so perplexing at first glance because they are unexpected. Furthermore, observations about the periodic formation of pre-cipitates in tinctures etc., as they originate spontaneously during the aging pro-cess of the system are to be found in Lloyd's treatise; also experimental and theoretical analysis of these observations is directly relevant to the analogous processes in gelatins. Moreover, J. U. Lloyd has described very interesting ex-periments with capillary analysis, apparently completely independently of the well-known experiments of Schönbein and F. Goppelsroeder etc. Here, experi-ments are described that treat one aspect of these events which has received relatively little attention. Systematic experiments are cited concerning the in-fluence of the concentration of dissolved substances, in respect to the level of pure water as well as to that of the dissolved material retained by the filter paper, etc. Here too, J. U. Lloyd describes thoroughly rigorous experiments. The pub-lisher knows of no more rigorous demonstration of the separation of adsorp-tion in capillary analysis than that of J. U. Lloyd, in which pure water (naturally, only in small quantities) is "pumped off" so to speak, not only from iron sul-fate solution, but also from diluted sulfuric acid by means of a strip of filter paper.

Previously, it has not been customary to include reprintings of treatises in the "Kolloid-Zeitschrift" and in the "Kolloidchemischen Beiheften." The publisher is of the opinion, however, that the majority of readers will agree with him, after studying Lloyd's treatise, that it constitutes a uniquely original contribution.

Wo. Ostwald

APPENDIX 4

The Significant Scientific Publications of John Uri Lloyd

Note: An asterisk before the date designates an Ebert Prize winner.

1874   "To What Do Our Plants Owe Their Value?" *Eclectic Medical Journal* 34 (December): 551–53.

1875   "Pharmaceutical Chemistry." *Electic Medical Journal* 35–36 (January 1875–August 1876). Comprises nine serialized articles.

1875   "Pharmaceutical Trifles." *Eclectic Medical Journal* 35 (February): 100–101.

1879   "On the Conditions Necessary to Successfully Conduct Percolation." *Proceedings of the American Pharmaceutical Association* 27: 682–705.

1880   With John King. *Supplement to the American Dispensatory.* Cincinnati: Wilstach, Baldwin.

1881   "Precipitates in Fluid Extracts." *Proceedings of the American Pharmaceutical Association* 29: 408–21.

1881   *The Chemistry of Medicines.* Cincinnati: Robert Clarke. Published in eight editions to 1897.

★1882   "Precipitates in Fluid Extracts." *Proceedings of the American Pharmaceutical Association* 30: 509–18.

1883   "Precipitates in Fluid Extracts." *Proceedings of the American Pharmaceutical Association* 31: 336–46.

1883   *Elixirs, Their History, Formulae, and Methods of Preparation.* Cincinnati: Robert Clarke. Also published as *Pharmaceutical Preparations: Elixirs, Their History, Formulae, and Methods of Preparation* in 1885; and as *Elixirs and Flavoring Extracts* in 1892 by William Wood.

1884   *Drugs and Medicines of North America: A Quarterly Devoted to the Historical and Scientific Discussion of Botany, Pharmacy, Chemistry and Therapeutics of the Medical Plants of North America.* Cincinnati: Lloyd Library. Two volumes were published, suspended in June of 1887. Also reissued as Bulletins 29–31. Cincinnati: Lloyd Library, 1930–1931.

1884   "Precipitates in Fluid Extracts." *Proceedings of the American Pharmaceutical Association* 32, 410–19.

1885   "Precipitates in Fluid Extracts." *Proceedings of the American Pharmaceutical Association* 33, 411–19.

1886   With John King. *The American Dispensatory*. Cincinnati: Wilstach, Baldwin. Lloyd also collaborated on the 1889, 1891, and 1895 editions.

1887   "Polypharmacy." *Eclectic Medical Journal* 47 (February): 70–72.

★1891   "Remarks Concerning a Scheme to Establish a Comparative Standard for Alkaloidal Galenics." *Proceedings of the American Pharmaceutical Association* 39, 124–33.

1898   With Harvey Wickes Felter. *King's American Dispensatory*. Cincinnati: Ohio Valley. Lloyd also collaborated on the 1905 and 1909 editions. Reprint, Sandy, OR: Eclectic Medical Publications, 1983.

1902   *References to Capillarity to the End of the Year 1900*. Bulletin 4. Cincinnati: Lloyd Library.

1910   *The Eclectic Alkaloids, Resins, Resinoids, Oleo-Resins and Concentrated Principles*. Bulletin 12. Cincinnati: Lloyd Library.

1915   With Finley Ellingwood. *American Materia Medica, Therapeutics, and Pharmacognosy*. Chicago: Ellingwood's Therapeutist. Lloyd also collaborated on a 1919 edition.

★1916   "Discovery of the Alkaloidal Affinities of Hydrous Aluminum Silicate." *Journal of the American Pharmaceutical Association* 5 (April): 381–90; 490–95.

1916   "Pharmazeutische Studien." *Kolloidchemische Beihefte* bd. 8, hft. 6–7: 171–250.

1921   *Origin and History of All the Pharmacopeial Vegetable Drugs*. Washington, DC: American Drug Manufacturer's Association. Reprint, Cincinnati: Caxton Press, 1929.

APPENDIX 5

Lloyd's Examinations at the EMI

The following are two examples of the exams given by John Uri Lloyd to medical students at the Eclectic Medical Institute.

SENIOR EXAMINATION
Chemistry and Pharmacy
John Uri Lloyd   May 31, 1894

1. What is the difference between (*a*) *prepared chalk* and (*b*) *precipitated chalk*?

2. What is understood by (*a*) valence; (*b*) fluorescence; (*c*) ebullition; (*d*) a precipitate; (*e*) amorphous?

3. Why should (*a*) potassium acetate be kept in a closely stoppered container? (*b*) Why should ammonium carbonate?

4. Describe ammonium chloride, and give its common name.

5. What is the difference between *ammonia* and *ammonium*?

6. How should you antidote (*a*) bromine vapor; (*b*) lead salts; (*c*) corrosive sublimate; (*d*) arsenic?

7. Name and describe a sublimate?

8. What color are the ferric salts, usually?

9. What is (*a*) copperas; (*b*) blue stone; (*c*) white precipitate; (*d*) Glauber's salt; (*e*) Epsom salt; (*f*) Rochelle salt?

10. How would you remove (*a*) fresh nitrate of silver stains; (*b*) iron stains?

11. Describe (*a*) magnesium carbonate; (*b*) zinc sulphate; (*c*) bismuth subnitrate?

12. How would you prepare mucilage of slippery elm?

13. How would you prepare spirit of Mindererus?

14. How would you prepare peppermint water?

15. What is the usual base of (*a*) a liniment; (*b*) an ointment; (*c*) a cerate; (*d*) a plaster?

16. What is lunar caustic?

17. What is liquor calcis?

18. What is (*a*) Lugol's solution; (*b*) Donovan's solution; (*c*) Fowler's solution?

19. What per cent of arsenical salt (or of arsenic) is in such of the foregoing substances as contain that substance?

20. What is (*a*) amylum; (*b*) adeps?

21. What is the chief difference between a fluid extract and a tincture?

JUNIOR EXAMINATION
Chemistry
John Uri Lloyd   May 30, 1894

1. Define an oxidizer.

2. Give the chemical name of (*a*) cream of tartar; (*b*) baking soda; (*c*) sal soda; (*d*) nitre; (*e*) Chili saltpeter.

3. What is the rule regarding the formation of (*a*) *ide* salts; (*b*) *ate* salts; (*c*) *ite* salts?

4. What is an (*a*) atom; (*b*) a molecule; (*c*) a symbol; (*d*) a formula; (*e*) an equation?

5. (*a*) Name and (*b*) describe two organic salts.

6. What is (*a*) a sulphate; (*b*) a sulphite; (*c*) a citrate?

7. What is the common name of ammonium chloride?

8. What is the antidote to caustic potash?

9. (*a*) Which is yellow, the cyanide or ferrocyanide of potassium? (*b*) Which is poisonous?

10. Describe (*a*) potassium acetate; (*b*) potassium permanganate; (*c*) sodium bicarbonate.

11. What will remove iodine stains?

12. Which of the following substances are elements: Sulphur, iodine, bromine, argols, saltpeter, sodium, argentum, aurum, niter.

13. What is the physical condition of each substance named in question 12?

Notes

Frequently cited sources are identified by the following abbreviations:

AIHP   American Institute of the History of Pharmacy
EMJ   *Eclectic Medical Journal*
J APhA   *Journal of the American Pharmaceutical Association*
KRF   Kremers Reference Files, F. B. Power Pharmaceutical Library, University
of Wisconsin
LLM   Lloyd Library and Museum, Cincinnati
NF   *The National Formulary*
Proceedings   *Proceedings of the American Pharmaceutical Association*
USD   *The United States Dispensatory*
USP   *The Pharmacopeia of the United States of America*

1. Lloyd's Early Years, 1849–1863

1. The booklet was apparently sent to Lloyd's mother by Hall's son years later. See LLM, coll. 8, box 1, folder 19.

2. On Lloyd's paternal ancestry, see Eunice A. Lloyd's recollections in LLM, coll. 1, box 3, folder 40.

3. Bruce Bliven Jr., *New York: A History* (New York: W. W. Norton, 1981), 83.

4. LLM, col. 8, box 1, folder 19.

5. Bliven, *New York*, 91.

6. For details, see Sophia Webster Lloyd's typescript, "Settlement on the Mohawk," LLM, coll. 8, box 1, folder 15.

7. See John Uri Lloyd's typescript fragment, LLM, coll. 8, box 1, folder 15.

8. John Uri Lloyd, "A Pharmaceutical Apprenticeship in America Fifty Years Ago," *J APhA* 4 (November 1915): 1333–34.

9. For details on Boone County growth, see Wendell H. Rone, *An Historical Atlas of Kentucky and Her Counties* (Central City, KY: W. Sandefur, 1965), 46–47.

10. LLM, coll. 1, box, folder 29.

11. See "Charles Green Land Journal, 1844–1892," in Susan S. Kissel and Margery T. Rouse, eds., *The Story of the Pewter Basin and Other Occasional Writings Collected in Southern Ohio and Northern Kentucky* (Bloomington, IN: T.I.S. Publications, 1981), 18.

12. Details on Emma's life are absent from the LLM archives. Surviving letters from both Curtis Gates and John Uri Lloyd's papers indicate a close relationship in which each referred to the other as "brother" and "sister." Extant correspondence shows that, even after marrying John D. Nead and moving to Kansas City, Missouri, Mrs. Emma Nead kept an active interest in Lloyd family affairs.

13. This cannot be confirmed in any of the extant LLM archival materials. The story is told in Corinne Miller Simons, *John Uri Lloyd, His Life and His Works, 1849–1936, with a History of the Lloyd Library* (Cincinnati: C. M. Simons, 1972), 13. Mrs. Simons was librarian at the Lloyd Library for more than thirty years and may have acquired some of her information from conversations with John Thomas Lloyd, John Uri's son. While Simons insists that the mustard plaster incident left a strong impression in the mind of John Uri Lloyd to fight for better treatment and better drug standards, there is no way to substantiate this from her undocumented book. If true, it surely would have remained a strong motivating factor for Lloyd to crusade for greater controls on all pharmaceuticals including patent medicines, but Lloyd's own silence on a matter so close to him personally makes the story suspect.

14. Daniel E. Sutherland states that more than 90 percent of Americans in the period had lost some family member by age fifteen. See *The Expansion of Everyday Life, 1860–1876* (New York: Harper & Row, 1989), 127.

15. Lloyd, "A Pharmaceutical Apprenticeship," 1333–41.

16. Lloyd, "A Pharmaceutical Apprenticeship," 1334–35.

17. Quoted in Reginald C. McGrane, *The Cincinnati Doctor's Forum* (Cincinnati: Academy of Medicine of Cincinnati, 1957), 9–10.

18. John Duffy, *From Humors to Medical Science: A History of American Medicine*, 2nd ed. (Urbana: University of Illinois Press, 1993), 150.

19. Duffy, *From Humors to Medical Science*, 182.

20. See Henry A. Ford and Kate B. Ford, *History of Cincinnati Ohio, with Illustrations and Biographical Sketches* (Cleveland: L. A. Williams, 1881; Cincinnati: Ohio Book Store, 1987), 172–202, 224–28, 323–24; and S. B. Nelson and J. M. Runk, *History of Cincinnati and Hamilton County, Ohio: Their Past and Present* (Cincinnati: S. B. Nelson, 1894), 96–155.

21. Ford and Ford, *History of Cincinnati*, 224.

22. Barry W. Bobst, "Agricultural and Mechanical College," in *The Kentucky Encyclopedia*, ed. John E. Kleber (Lexington: University Press of Kentucky, 1992), 5–6.

23. On the centralization and standardization of education in America, see Donald R. Warren, *To Enforce Education: A History of the Founding Years of the United States Office of Education* (Detroit: Wayne State University Press, 1974).

24. LLM, coll. 1, box 2, folder 9.

25. Letter from Edward Webster to John Uri Lloyd, July 17, 1869, LLM, coll. 1, box 6, folder 63.

26. For details, see *Kremers and Urdang's History of Pharmacy*, 4th ed., rev. by Glenn Sonnedecker (Philadelphia: J. B. Lippincott, 1976; reprint, Madison, WI: AIHP, 1986), 226–54.

27. Sonnedecker, *History of Pharmacy*, 244.

28. *Fourth Annual Announcement of the Cincinnati College of Pharmacy, Session 1874–1875* (Cincinnati: Bradley & Power, 1874). Although an earlier Cincinnati College of Pharmacy was chartered by the state legislature on March 23, 1850, it ceased operations with the advent of the Civil War.

29. Sonnedecker, *History of Pharmacy*, 244.

30. With the fall of Vicksburg on July 4, 1863, the entire trans-Mississippi and Ohio

waterways were secured under Union control, thus becoming a critical artery in supplying Union troops in the western theater.

31. LLM, coll. 1, box 2, folder 9.

2. THE RUSTIC APPRENTICE, 1864–1870

1. Daniel Hurley, *Cincinnati, the Queen City* (Cincinnati: Cincinnati Historical Society, 1982), 76.

2. See Friedrich Ratzel's description in his *Sketches of Urban and Cultural Life in North America*, trans. and ed. Stewart A. Stehlin (New Brunswick, NJ: Rutgers University Press, 1988), 230–236.

3. For details on German immigration at this time, see Hurley, *Cincinnati*, 44–46.

4. Sutherland, *Expansion of Everyday Life*, x.

5. A biographical sketch can be found in Lloyd, "A Pharmaceutical Apprenticeship," 1342.

6. John Uri Lloyd, "Activities of W. J. M. Gordon," *EMJ* 86 (November 1926): 1–4.

7. Lloyd, "A Pharmaceutical Apprenticeship," 1335.

8. For details, see J. F. Hancock, "Reminiscences Pharmaceutical," *Druggists Circular* 51 (January 1907): 181–83.

9. See wage figures in Sutherland, *Expansion of Everyday Life*, 134, 168.

10. Teresa Catherine Gallagher, "From Helpmeet to Independent Professional: Women in American Pharmacy, 1870–1940," *Pharmacy in History* 31 (1989): 60–77.

11. Sonnedecker, *History of Pharmacy*, 291.

12. Sonnedecker, *History of Pharmacy*, 214–19.

13. For details, see Sonnedecker, *History of Pharmacy*, chapter 15, especially pp. 282–89.

14. Procter's contributions to pharmacy are given full treatment in Gregory J. Higby, *In Service to American Pharmacy: The Professional Life of William Procter, Jr.* (Tuscaloosa: University of Alabama Press, 1992).

15. On the early development of the *USP*, see Glenn Sonnedecker's three-part study, "The Founding Period of the U.S. Pharmacopeia," *Pharmacy in History* 35 (1993): 151–62; 36 (1994): 3–25; and 36 (1994): 103–22.

16. Lee Anderson and Gregory Higby, *The Spirit of Voluntarism: A Legacy of Commitment and Contribution: The United States Pharmacopeia, 1820–1995* (Rockville, MD: USP Convention, 1995), 85.

17. Anderson and Higby, *The Spirit of Voluntarism*, 53.

18. Anderson and Higby, *The Spirit of Voluntarism*, 55.

19. Lloyd, "A Pharmaceutical Apprenticeship," 1334.

20. Lloyd, "A Pharmaceutical Apprenticeship," 1338.

21. Lloyd, "A Pharmaceutical Apprenticeship," 1335.

22. J. F. Hancock, "Early Detroit Stores," *Druggists Circular* 51 (January 1907): 188.

23. A. E. Magoffin, "Recollections of an Old-Time Druggist," *Druggists Circular* 51 (January 1907): 192–93.

24. Lloyd, "A Pharmaceutical Apprenticeship," 1339.

25. Sutherland, *Expansion of Everyday Life*, 28, 97.

26. See Diary entries in LLM, coll. 1, box 1, folders 1, 2, and 4.

27. Letter dated March 28, 1868, LLM, coll. 8, box 1, folder 2.

28. John Uri Lloyd, "Fragments from an Autobiography. My Entrance into Eclectic Pharmacy," *EMJ* 87 (July 1927): 303–11. Lloyd stated that King made this offer in 1870, but the date must be incorrect. It must be remembered that Lloyd was writing (probably from memory) more than fifty years after these events occured. Given the evidence in his own diary written at the time, the Lloyd brothers would hardly have been launching a business of their own in late 1870, with King's offer for John to join H. M. Merrell still outstanding. More than likely, King made his proposition in early 1871.

3. The Lure of Eclecticism

1. W. F. Bynum, *Science and the Practice of Medicine in the Nineteenth Century* (New York: Cambridge University Press, 1994), 219.

2. Abraham Flexner, *Medical Education in the United States and Canada: A Report to the Carnegie Foundation for the Advancement of Teaching*, Bulletin 4 (New York: Carnegie Foundation, 1910), 156.

3. The original 1822 edition is now quite scarce. Lloyd recognized Thomson as a significant force in promoting an indigenous plant materia medica and reproduced a later 1825 printing of *The New Guide to Health* as Bulletin of the Lloyd Library of Botany, Pharmacy and Materia Medica 11. Reproduction Series 7 (Cincinnati: LLM, 1909).

4. The most thorough modern treatment of Thomsonianism to date is available in Alex Berman, *The Thomsonian Movement and Its Relation to American Pharmacy and Medicine*, Contributions from the History of Pharmacy Department of the School of Pharmacy, University of Wisconsin, no. 2 (Madison: AIHP, 1952); a briefer account of Thomsonianism is available in Susan E. Fillmore, "Samuel Thomson and His Effect on the American Health Care System," *Pharmacy in History* 28 (1986): 188–91.

5. Letter from Samuel Thomson to R. K. Frost, December 9, 1837. Original in the rare book room of LLM.

6. Alex Berman, "Neo-Thomsonianism in the United States," *Journal of the History of Medicine and Allied Sciences* 11 (1956): 133–55.

7. The eclectics did try to associate themselves with the French eclectic movement and even with classical antiquity. See Vincent Millasich, "Eclecticism and Its Origin," *California Eclectic Medical Journal* 6 (December 1913): 299–301; and Alexander Wilder, *History of Medicine* (Augusta, ME: Maine Farmer Publishing, 1904), 91, 212. But such claims were strained and stemmed more from polemical rhetoric than from historical fact. American eclectics and French eclectics, for example, shared little more than the vernacular sense of the name. René Laennec (1781–1826), the first to apply Victor Cousin's term "eclectic" to his philosophy of medicine, was an extreme Royalist, which made him a well paid but unpopular physician and delayed his recognition as the greatest of French clinicians until modern times. Later, Gabriel Andral (1791–1876), considered a pioneer in hematology and laboratory medicine, led the movement of medical eclecticism in France. Frédéric Bérard (1789–1828), professor of public health at the Faculté de Médecine, headed a Montepellier group of eclectics. Whatever their philosophical tenets, no amount of argument by eclectics on American soil could discount the fact that (unlike themselves) Laennec, Andral, and Bérard were all recognized members of the medical establishment. For more on the French eclectic movement, see the following: Erwin H. Ackerknecht, *Medicine at the Paris Hospital, 1794–1848* (Baltimore: Johns Hopkins Uni-

versity Press, 1967), 101–13; Jacalyn Duffin, "Private Practice and Public Research: The Patients of R. T. H. Laennec," in *French Medical Culture in the Nineteenth Century*, ed. Ann La Berge and Mordechai Feingold (Amsterdam: Rodopi, 1994), 118–48; and Elizabeth A. Williams, *The Physical and the Moral: Anthropology, Physiology, and Philosophical Medicine in France, 1750–1850* (New York: Cambridge University Press, 1994), 140–51.

8. Alex Berman, "The Heroic Approach In 19th Century Therapeutics," *Bulletin, American Society of Hospital Pharmacy* (September–October 1954): 319–27.

9. The most complete, objective history of the eclectics is John S. Haller Jr., *Medical Protestants: The Eclectics in American Medicine, 1825–1939* (Carbondale: Southern Illinois University Press, 1994). The allusion to Protestantism is drawn from Dr. Edward B. Foote, a New York eclectic physician.

10. John Milton Scudder, "The Essential Difference Between the Three Schools of Medicine: Allopathic, Eclectic, and Homeopathic," *EMJ* 69 (January 1909): 10.

11. Quoted in Alex Berman, "Wooster Beach and the Early Eclectics," *University of Michigan Medical Bulletin* 24 (July 1958): 281.

12. On early eclectic medical schools, see the summary in Haller, *Medical Protestants*, 75–84.

13. Harvey Wickes Felter, *History of the Eclectic Medical Institute* (Cincinnati: Alumnal Association of the Eclectic Medical Institute, 1902), 30.

14. Ronald L. Numbers, "The Making of an Eclectic Physician: Joseph M. McElhinney and the Eclectic Medical Institute of Cincinnati," *Bulletin of the History of Medicine* 47 (March–April 1973): 160.

15. Haller, *Medical Protestants*, 216.

16. Numbers, "Making of an Eclectic Physician," 166.

17. Berman, "Wooster Beach," 282–83.

18. John King, "Eclectic Pharmacopoeia," *EMJ* 30 (September 1870): 435–36.

19. Lloyd, "Fragments from an Autobiography," 304.

20. For details on the William S. Merrell firm, see the company history commemorating its 125th anniversary, by Alice Van Pelt, *Since 1828* (Cincinnati: William S. Merrell, 1953).

21. Felter, *History of the Eclectic Medical Institute*, 78.

22. Wilder, *History of Medicine*, 659.

23. John King, editorial, *Western Medical Reformer* 5 (April 1846): 176.

24. Alex Berman, "The Eclectic 'Concentrations' and American Pharmacy (1847–1861)," *Pharmacy in History* 22 (1980): 91–103.

25. Quoted in Berman, "The Eclectic 'Concentrations,'" 92.

26. G. W. L. Bickley, "Concentration of Medicines," *EMJ* 1, series 5 (February 1857): 68–71.

27. Robert S. Newton, "Concentration of Medicines," *EMJ* 1, series 5 (March 1857): 144–45.

28. Walter Miller Ingalls, "Concentrated Remedies," *EMJ* 1, series 4 (September 1856): 413.

29. Quoted in Higby, *In Service to American Pharmacy*, 7–8.

30. Quoted in Berman, "The Eclectic 'Concentrations,'" 95.

31. John King, "Concentrated Medicines Adulterated," *Worcester Journal of Medicine* 10 (June 1855): 225–27.

32. This divisive period is discussed at length in Haller, *Medical Protestants*, 119–22.

33. Edwin S. Wayne, "Criticism of the Value of Concentrated Preparations," *College Journal of Medical Science* 1 (February 1856): 45–48.

34. William S. Merrell, "Reply of Mr. Merrell," *College Journal of Medical Science* 1 (February 1856): 48–49.

35. King, "Concentrated Medicines Adulterated," 225–27. Lloyd gives the historical context of King's comments in his *Eclectic Alkaloids, Resins, Resinoids, Oleo-Resins and Concentrated Principles*, Bulletin of the Lloyd Library of Botany, Pharmacy and Materia Medica 12 (Cincinnati: LLM, 1910), 33. It should be mentioned in passing that Merrell's 1856 price list shows "Jalapin" selling for precisely $1 per ounce (see p. 28). A briefer account of the eclectic concentration controversy is given in Lloyd, *A Treatise on the American Alkaloids, Resins, Oleo-Resins and Concentrated Principles (so-called Eclectic Concentrations)*, Drug Treatise 24 (Cincinnati: Lloyd Brothers, 1909).

36. Lloyd, *The Eclectic Alkaloids*, 18.

37. John King, "Mr. Merrell and His Manufactures," *College Journal of Medical Science* 1 (March 1856): 90–92.

38. See John King, *American Dispensatory*, 5th ed. (Cincinnati: Moore, Wilstach, Keys, 1859), xii. King's praise of Wayne was carried in all subsequent editions until an entirely new preface was added to the 18th edition, with Harvey Wickes Felter and John Uri Lloyd's collaboration in 1898.

39. Lloyd, *The Eclectic Alkaloids*, 45–50.

40. Lloyd, *The Eclectic Alkaloids*, 41.

41. Lloyd, "Fragments from an Autobiography," 304.

42. Scudder's ideas are summarized in Haller, *Medical Protestants*, 176–83.

43. John Milton Scudder, *Specific Medication and Specific Medicines* (Cincinnati: Wilstach, Baldwin, 1870).

44. Scudder, *Specific Medication*, 32–33.

45. Lloyd Brothers, *Dose Book of Specific Medicines* (Cincinnati: Lloyd Brothers, 1907), 11.

46. Lloyd, "Fragments from an Autobiography," 305.

47. The *Eclectic Medical Journal* for 1870 ran consistent ads listng William S. Merrell and Company, H. M. Merrell and Company, T. L. A. Greve, and J. F. Judge as providers of "Specific Medicine." By 1872, however, H. M. Merrell was the only wholesaler advertising these medicines.

48. See table 5.1 in Haller, *Medical Protestants*, 164–165.

49. Frederick C. Waite, "Thomsonianism in Ohio," *Ohio State Archaeological and Historical Quarterly* 49 (October–December 1940): 329.

50. Lloyd, "Fragments from an Autobiography," 307.

51. For details on King and Scudder, see John Uri Lloyd, *Biographies of John King, M.D., Andrew Jackson Howe, A.B., M.D., and John Milton Scudder, M.D.* Bulletin of the Lloyd Library of Botany, Pharmacy and Materia Medica 19 (Cincinnati: LLM, 1912), 3–110, and 237–355.

52. Otto Juettner, *Daniel Drake and His Followers, 1785–1909* (Cincinnati: Harvey Publishing, 1909), 371.

53. Lloyd, *Biographies of King, Howe, and Scudder*, 8.

54. See the following Lloyd articles in the *EMJ*: "Eclectic Pharmacopoeia" (October 1870–January 1871); "To What Do Our Medicinal Plants Owe Their Value?" (December 1874): 551–553; "Pharmaceutical Chemistry" (January 1875–August 1876);

"Pharmaceutical Trifles" (February 1875): 100–101; "Note on Salicylic Acid" (August 1875): 366–368; "Euphorbia Hypericifolia" (September 1875): 409–410; "Grindela Robusta" (February 1876): 67–70; "Gelsemium Sempervirens" (March 1876): 105–12; "Chlorophyll and Medicine" (April 1876): 163–65; "Eriodyction Glutinosum" (May 1876): 247–248; "Tinctures Made From Fresh Herbs" (June 1876): 260–62; "Green Tinctures" (July 1876): 310–14; "Diseases From Soap" (September–October 1876): 400–402, 454–456; "Fluid Extract of Gossypium Herbaceum" (December 1876): 538–47.

55. Information on the Lloyd brothers' early business activities can be found in "Evolution of the House of Lloyd Brothers," LLM, coll. 1, box 2, folder 14.

56. "Addie Meader Lloyd," LLM, coll. 1, box 2, folders 33–34.

4. BUSY WITH BUSINESS: FROM MERRELL, THORP, AND LLOYD TO LLOYD BROTHERS

1. See LLM, coll. 1, box 6, folder 72; box 12, folders 256–262; box 9, folder 181; and box 11, folder 245.

2. See, for example, his letter of March 4, 1896, to his mother, LLM, coll. 1, box 6, folder 56.

3. Alfred L. Thimm, *Business Ideologies in the Reform-Progressive Era, 1880–1914* (Tuscaloosa: University of Alabama Press, 1976), 9–10.

4. Thimm, *Business Ideologies,* 4.

5. Richard B. Morris, ed., *Encyclopedia of American History* (New York: Harper & Row, 1976), 748.

6. Morris, *Encyclopedia of American History,* 775.

7. David L. Cowen and William H. Helfand, *Pharmacy: An Illustrated History* (New York: Harry N. Abrams, 1990), 124; see also David L. Cowen, "The Role of the Pharmaceutical Industry," in *Safeguarding the Public: Historical Aspects of Medicinal Drug Control* (Baltimore: Johns Hopkins University Press, 1970), 72–82.

8. Anderson and Higby, *The Spirit of Voluntarism,* 215.

9. For details, see part II of Joseph P. Remington, *The Practice of Pharmacy,* 1st ed. (Philadelphia: J. B. Lippincott, 1885), 245–397.

10. Remington, *Practice of Pharmacy,* 1st ed., 325–26.

11. Sonnedecker, *History of Pharmacy,* 331.

12. Charles L. Huisking, *Herbs to Hormones: The Evolution of Drugs and Chemicals that Revolutionized Medicine* (Essex, CT: Pequot Press, 1968), 36.

13. Patent medicines have been the subject of several interesting studies. See, for example, James Harvey Young, *Toadstool Millionaires* (Princeton, NJ: Princeton University Press, 1961); J. Worth Estes, "'Shaker-Made' Remedies," *Pharmacy in History* 34 (1992): 63–73; George B. Griffenhagen and James Harvey Young, "Old English Patent Medicines," *Pharmacy in History* 34 (1992): 200–29; and Varro E. Tyler, "Was Lydia E. Pinkham's Vegetable Compound an Effective Remedy?," *Pharmacy in History* 37 (1995): 24–28.

14. Sonnedecker, *History of Pharmacy,* 325.

15. Haller, *Medical Protestants,* 182.

16. See advertisements in *EMJ* 38 (January 1878): 9; and *EMJ* 38 (February 1878): 3–7.

17. The troy ounce had become the official pharmacopeial standard of apothecary weight with the sanction of the committee of revision of *USP* IV in 1860; see Anderson

and Higby, *The Spirit of Voluntarism*, 82. 1 troy ounce = 480 grains; 12 troy ounces = 1 pound (5,760 grains).

18. See 1879 Parke, Davis and Company price list in LLM, special coll. 101, box 67, folder 1.

19. See Thorp and Lloyd Brothers' catalogs, LLM, coll. 6, box 5, folder 25.

20. See John Uri Lloyd, "Experiments upon Dilute Hydrocyanic Acid," *Proceedings* 25 (1877): 695–99.

21. "Report on the Committee on Exhibition," *Proceedings* 29 (1881): 397–98.

22. William S. Merrell, "The Fluid Extracts of Wm. S. Merrell & Co. and Their Relation to the So-called 'Specific Medicines,'" LLM, coll. 6, box 9, folder 129.

23. *Thorp & Lloyd Brothers' Complete Physicians' Catalogue*, LLM, coll. 6, box 5, folder 25.

24. Compare with standards for fluidextracts specified for each item in *USP*, 6th dec. rev. ed. (New York: William Wood, 1882), 122, 121, 143, 144, 146.

25. Scudder, *Specific Medication*, 32.

26. Lloyd Brothers, *Dose Book*, 7–8.

27. John Uri Lloyd, "Specific Medicines are Definite," *EMJ* 36 (November 1876): 503–504.

28. See Lloyd Brothers, *Dose Book*, LLM, coll. 6, boxes 3–4, folders 9–22.

29. Scudder, *Specific Medication*, 33.

30. John Uri Lloyd, "On the Use of Fresh and Dry Plants for Tinctures," *Proceedings* 26 (1878): 755–56.

31. See advertisements in *EMJ* 45 (November 1885): 5–8.

32. Jonathan Liebenau, *Medical Science and Medical Industry: The Formation of the American Pharmaceutical Industry* (Baltimore: Johns Hopkins University Press, 1987), 32.

33. Liebenau, *Medical Science and Medical Industry*, 5.

34. Alex Berman, "A Striving for Scientific Respectability: Some American Botanics and the Nineteenth-Century Plant Materia Medica," *Bulletin of the History of Medicine* 30 (January–February 1956): 7–31.

5. "The Wizard of American Plant Pharmacy and Chemistry": John Uri Lloyd in His Laboratory

1. James H. Beal, "Some Aspects of Eclecticisim as They Appear to a Majority of Pharmacists," *EMJ* 91 (November 1931): 436.

2. *Dictionary of Scientific Biography*, ed. Charles Coulston Gillispie (New York: Charles Scribner's, 1973), 8:427–28.

3. "List of Queries," *Proceedings* 27 (1879): 15.

4. John Uri Lloyd, "On the Conditions Necessary to Successfully Conduct Percolation," *Proceedings* 27 (1879): 682–708.

5. The exact processes of percolation involve the activities of gravity, downward displacement, and hydrostatic pressure, whereby a suitable solvent passes through a column of plant drug contained in a percolator and dissolves or extracts the desired chemical agents contained within the cell of the powdered drug. The author is thankful to Patrick F. Belcastro, a professor emeritus of pharmaceutics at Purdue University, for this observation.

6. Although frequently considered a uniquely American contribution to pharmacy,

percolation did not originate in the United States. Procter's work on percolation beginning in the mid-1840s was preceeded by François Réal's preliminary work in 1816, J. A. Buchner's contributions in 1822, and Pierre and Polydore Boulay's studies on "nonpressure displacement" in 1833. For details, see Milton Wruble, "Studies in Percolation," *American Journal of Pharmacy* 105 (May 1933): 244–47; (June 1933): 289–295; and (July 1933): 340–52.

7. This is an admittedly descriptive rather than precise definition of colloids. Today colloids would be defined by pharmaceutical researchers more quantitatively. Dr. Belcastro offers the following modern definition: "A dispersion in which the dissolved particles are in the form of small molecules or ions are *true solutions* and the size of these ions or molecules is usually less than 10 Angstroms (A). Dispersed particles are in the *colloidal* range when the size is between 10A and 0.5 micron. In a *course dispersion* (suspensions for example) the particle size ranges from ½ micron to 100 microns in diameter." Even by this more modern definition, Belcastro agrees that "the percolates coming out a percolator do indeed contain colloidal material." Letter from Patrick F. Belcastro to the author, March 3–4, 1996.

8. Cowen and Helfand, *Pharmacy*, 113.

9. For details on the development of colloidal theory, see Sir William Cecil Dampier, *A History of Science*, 3rd ed. (New York: Cambridge University Press, 1946), 266, 280–81, 359–60.

10. Precipitates are by definition materials that settle out of a solution or suspension medium either by the forces of gravity or chemical reaction. The chemical symbol (↓) is as descriptive as it is indicative of the process.

11. See Lloyd's series of articles titled "Precipitates in Fluid Extracts": *Proceedings* 29 (1881): 408–21; *Proceedings* 30 (1882): 502–18; *Proceedings* 31 (1883): 336–46; *Proceedings* 32 (1884): 410–19; and *Proceedings* 33 (1885): 411–19.

12. Lloyd, "Precipitates," *Proceedings* 29 (1881): 409. As Lloyd would eventually discover, precipitates are not necessarily objectionable. Colloidal dust particles such as coal and soot in a closed environment, for example, can be eliminated from the atmosphere by introducing an opposite electrical charge, thus forcing the material to precipitate down and out of the air. Lloyd would find that the application of this general principle to pharmacy would hold special significance.

13. Lloyd, "Precipitates," *Proceedings* 29 (1881): 421.

14. Lloyd, "Precipitates," *Proceedings* 32 (1884): 419.

15. John Uri Lloyd, "Remarks Concerning a Scheme to Establish a Comparative Standard for Alkaloidal Galenicals," *Proceedings* 39 (1891): 124–33.

16. John Uri Lloyd, "Discovery of the Alkaloidal Affinities of Hydrous Aluminum Silicate," *J APhA* 5 (April 1916): 381–90, 490–495.

17. For a fascinating account of the historical uses of plants in this and other contexts, see John Mann, *Murder, Magic, and Medicine* (New York: Oxford University Press, 1994).

18. For a thorough discussion of the discovery of alkaloids, see John Lesch, "Conceptual Changes in an Empirical Science: The Discovery of the First Alkaloids," *Historical Studies in the Physical Sciences* 11 (1981): 305–28.

19. John Uri Lloyd, "Remarks on Lloyd's Reagent," *J APhA* 3 (May 1914): 625–27.

20. The principles of adsorption have always been important in filtering processes since they involve the attraction of solid, liquid, or gaseous particles of one substance (e.g.,

alkaloids) to another (e.g., Lloyd's reagent). The ability of activated charcoal to adsorb substances nearly equal to its own weight explains its common application in air conditioner filters, dehumidifiers, and water treatment systems. In contrast to *absorption*, which involves the assimilation of particles *into* substances, in *adsorption* these particles are captured and carried *on the surface* of the adsorptive agent.

21. H. M. Gordon and Jay Kaplin, "Note on the Comparative Adsorption of Different Substances by Lloyd's Reagent, Animal Charcoal and Aluminum Hydroxide," *J APhA* 3 (May 1914): 627–30.

22. *Eclectic Review* 16 (December 1913); see also the *Bulletin of Pharmacy* 28 (January 1914): 3.

23. Bernard Fantus, "Fuller's Earth: Its Adsorptive Power, and Its Antidotal Value for Alkaloids," *Journal of the American Medical Association* 64 (May 29, 1915): 1838–1845. Today improved antagonists to narcotics such as naloxone hydrochloride have replaced these earlier remedies.

24. The ads ran in the *EMJ* 76 January through March of 1916.

25. See part I of the "Alphabetical Index to Pharmaceutical Specialties and Biologicals," in the *Physician's Desk Reference*, 10th ed. (Ordell, NJ: Medical Economics, 1955).

26. H. R. Rosenberg, *Chemistry and Physiology of the Vitamins* (New York: Interscience Publishers, 1942), 155–56. George Beal also made note of this in his "Lloyds of Cincinnati," *American Journal of Pharmaceutical Education* 23 (spring 1959): 204.

27. John Uri Lloyd, "Pharmazeutische Studien," *Kolloidchemische Beihefte*, bd. 8, hft. 6–7 (1916): 171–250. For details on the life of Ostwald, see *Dictionary of Scientific Biography*, 9:251–52.

28. Wolfgang Ostwald, "Vorbemerkung der Radaktion," *Kolloidchemische Beihefte*, bd. 8, hft. 6–7 (1916): 171–73. The author is grateful for the translation by Mary Jo Fasold and the assistance of Dr. Thomas H. Leech of Northern Kentucky University.

29. Wolfgang Ostwald, *An Introduction to Theoretical and Applied Colloid Chemistry*, trans. Martin H. Fischer (New York: J. Wiley, 1917), 119. The book was published in a second edition in 1922.

30. George Urdang, "The Scope of Pharmacy," *American Journal of Pharmaceutical Education* 9 (October 1945): 497.

31. Burkhard Reber, *Gallerie hervorragender Therapeutiker und Pharmakognosten der Gegenwart* (Geneva: Paul Dubois, 1894). A tranlsation of Reber's entry on Lloyd is available at the LLM. For more on Reber, see Lydia Mex, "Burkhard Reber: A Pharmacist-Collector and His Collection," *Pharmacy in History* 27 (1985): 90–95.

32. See *Dictionary of Scientific Biography*, 8:447–48.

33. See the bound presentation copy, *A Study in Pharmacy*, with typescript introduction in the LLM collection.

34. Remington, *Practice of Pharmacy*, 1st ed., 327.

35. See John Uri Lloyd, "Concentration of Low Temperature," *American Druggist* 17 (May 1888): 81; Lloyd, "What Is the Effect of Heat and Moisture as a Preparatory Step in the Extraction of Some Drugs," *Western Druggist* 11 (July 1889): 236; Lloyd, "Influences of Heat," *EMJ* 49 (January 1889): 27–29; and Lloyd, "The Influence of Heat and Moisture Upon Drugs," *Proceedings* 37 (1889): 79–84.

36. LLM, coll. 1, box 17, folder 323.

37. Letter from F. B. Kilmer to Frederick B. Power, June 10, 1909. LLM, coll. 1, box 17, folder 334 (carbon copy).

38. *Remington's Practice of Pharmacy*, 9th ed. (Easton, PA: Mack Publishing, 1948), 222.

39. See *Remington's Pharmaceutical Sciences*, 15th ed. (Easton, PA: Mack Publishing, 1975), 1517.

40. Lloyd's patents and related materials are located in LLM, coll. 1, box 17, folders 316–40.

41. Quoted in Neal Baldwin, *Edison: Inventing the Century* (New York: Hyperion, 1995), 86.

42. Baldwin, *Edison*, 25.

43. Baldwin, *Edison*, 41.

6. Building a Workshop: John Uri Lloyd and His Library

1. Quoted in Kenneth Brough, "The Heart of the University," in *Reader in American Library History*, ed. Michael H. Harris (Washington, DC: NCR Microcard, 1971), 214.

2. Lloyd, "The Founding of the Lloyd Library," *Proceedings* 52 (1904): 445–48; also published in *Pharmaceutical Review* 22 (October 1904): 357–61.

3. Walter Aiken, "Half Hours with the Lloyd Library," undated flier, LLM; Simons, *John Uri Lloyd*, 24; and Sigmund Waldbott, "The Lloyd Library," KRF, C36, c (I).

4. John Uri Lloyd, "Founding the Lloyd Library," *Proceedings* 52 (1904): 446.

5. Caswell A. Mayo, *The Lloyd Library and Its Makers*, Bulletin of the Lloyd Library of Botany, Pharmacy and Materia Medica 28 (Cincinnati: LLM, 1928), 17.

6. "An Interesting Letter from John Uri Lloyd," *Midland Druggist* 3 (February 1902): 525; also published as "Prof. Lloyd and the Lloyd Library," *Chicago Medical Times* 35 (January 1902): 85.

7. Letter from Lloyd to Kremers, March 12, 1903, KRF, A2, file 11.

8. Letter from Lloyd to Kremers, May 27, 1905, KRF, A2, file 12.

9. For details, see Corinne Miller Simons, "The Lloyd Library and Museum—A Brief History of Its Founders and Its Resources," *College and Research Libraries* 2 (June 1941): 2–4; and the classification at LLM.

10. For details, see Wayne Wiegand, "Dewey Declassified: A Revelatory Look at the 'Irrepressible Reformer,'" *American Libraries* 27 (January 1996): 54–60.

11. John Shaw Billings started work on the catalog in 1873, and by 1880 the first volume was issued as the *Index-Catalogue of the Library of the Surgeon-General's Office, United States Army* (Washington, DC: GPO, 1880). For details, see Michael H. Harris, *A History of Libraries in the Western World* (Metuchen, NJ: Scarecrow Press, 1984), 252; and Wyndam D. Miles, *A History of the National Library of Medicine: The Nation's Treasury of Medical Knowledge* (Washington, DC: GPO, 1982).

12. David Mearns, "The Library of Congress under Putnam," in Harris, ed., *Reader in American Library History*, 232–41.

13. Mayo, *The Lloyd Library*, 41.

14. See LLM, coll. 1, box 20, scrapbook 3.

15. LLM, coll. 1, box 25, scrapbook 10.

16. This assumes a 10 percent royalty with 40,000 out of the total 50,000 copies sold at $1.50 each.

17. See Thomas J. Schlereth, *Victorian America: Transformations in Everyday Life* (New York: Harper, 1991), 81.

18. John Uri Lloyd, "Prof. Lloyd," *Chicago Medical Times* 35 (January 1902): 85; and Lloyd, "An Interesting Letter," *Midland Druggist* 3 (February 1902): 525.

19. Letter from Lloyd to Kremers, September 29, 1905, KRF, A2, file 12.

20. Letter from Lloyd to Kremers, November 20, 1905, KRF, A2, file 12.

21. Letter from Lloyd to Kremers, April 6, 1909, KRF, A2, file 12.

22. Letter from Lloyd to Kremers, July 8, 1903, KRF, A2, file 11.

23. Letter from Provost Harrison to Lloyd, July 7, 1904, KRF, C36, c (I).

24. Letter from Oldberg to Lloyd, August 5, 1904, LLM.

25. Letter from Jenkins to Lloyd, October 3, 1904, KRF, C36, c (I).

26. Letter from Lloyd to Coville, October 3, 1904, KRF, C36, c (I).

27. Letter from Ebert to Lloyd, October 16, 1904, KRF, C36, c (I).

28. Letter from Lloyd to Kremers, October 1, 1909, KRF, A2, file 12.

29. Letter from Lloyd to Beal, March 7, 1910, KRF, A2, file 13.

30. Russel Manning, "John Uri Lloyd, Pharmaceutical Pathfinder, Wins Remington Honor Medal," *EMJ* 96 (1936): 188–90.

31. Felter, *History of the Eclectic Medical Institute*, 68–69.

32. Haller, *Medical Protestants*, 243; Eclectic Medical Institute Records, LLM, coll. 3, box 23, folders 685–92.

33. Mayo, *The Lloyd Library*, 47.

34. Print request form, LLM.

35. See Lloyd's offer and the committee's reply in *J APhA* 1 (October 1912): 1099, 1108.

36. Most of the Lloyd Library archives are part of the Curtis Gates Lloyd Papers, LLM, coll. 11, boxes 3–5.

37. LLM, coll. 11, box 5, folder 48.

38. Both documents are on display in the reading room of the Lloyd Library.

39. For details on the Walker papers, see Corinne Miller Simons, "Walker's Eclectic Collection in Lloyd Library," *National Eclectic Medical Quarterly* 41 (June 1950): 8–13.

40. See letters from John to Curtis, August 10, 1906, and January 15, 1907, LLM, coll. 11, box 10, folder 203.

41. Martin H. Fischer, "American Contemporaries—John Uri Lloyd," *EMJ* 96 (1936): 201–203.

42. See LLM, coll. 11, boxes 11–13.

43. George Urdang, *Pharmacy's Part in Society* (Madison, WI: AIHP, 1954), 37–38; Harris, *A History of Libraries*, 262; David Hoffman, *The Information Sourcebook of Herbal Medicine* (Freedom, CA: Crossing Press, 1994), 24–25; David M. Eisenberg, "Advising Patients Who Seek Alternative Medical Therapies," *Annals of Internal Medicine* 127 (July 1, 1997): 61–69.

44. See, for example, Mayo, *The Lloyd Library*, 24–31; and Simons, *John Uri Lloyd*, 123–30.

45. John Uri Lloyd, *Etidorhpa, or The End of Earth* (Cincinnati: Robert Clarke, 1895), v–vi.

7. Lloyd as Scholar

1. Glenn Sonnedecker, "American Pharmaceutical Historiography I," in *Pharmaceutical Historiography: Proceedings of a Colloquium Sponsored by the American Institute of the*

History of Pharmacy on the Occasion of the Institute's 25th Anniversary, Madison, Wisconsin, January 22–23, 1966, ed. Alex Berman (Madison: AIHP, 1967), 73.

2. See John Uri Lloyd, "Leisure Hours," *EMJ* 38 (July 1878): 305–307; Lloyd, "Organized Water as Food," *EMJ* 62 (September 1902): 596–600; and Lloyd, "The Ocean of Vitality and Reservoir of Life," *EMJ* 82 (January 1922): 1–3.

3. John Uri Lloyd, "An Investigator in Pharmacy—Historical," *EMJ* 85 (March 1925): 109–14.

4. John Uri Lloyd, "To What Do Our Medicinal Plants Owe Their Value?" *EMJ* 34 (December 1874): 551–53.

5. See, for example, the work of Friedrich W. A. Sertürner and Pierre Joseph Pelletier together with Joseph Bienaimé Caventou in extracting strychnine from nux vomica in 1818 and later (1820) quinine from cinchona; the publication of Nicolas J. B. G. Guibourt's influential *Histoire naturelle des drogues simples* in 1820; and the isolation of salicin from the willow by Johannes A. Buchner in 1828. In contrast, although William Procter, E. S. Wayne, R. H. Stabler, and J. M. Abernathy had pursued some phytochemical investigations, most work by American authors, such as Benjamin Smith Barton's *Collections for an Essay Towards a Materia Medica of the United States* (1798–1804), William P. C. Barton's *Vegetable Materia Medica of the United States* (1817–18), Constantine Rafinesque's *Medical Flora of the United States* (1828–30), and R. Eglesfeld Griffith's *Medical Botany* (1847), were all descriptive and empirical rather than analytic.

6. Sonnedecker, *History of Pharmacy*, 286.

7. John Uri Lloyd, "Pharmaceutical Trifles," *EMJ* 35 (February 1875): 100–101.

8. Some of the proprietary mixtures were even more flagrant in their conglomerations. But these can be found in the "Formulary of Unofficial Preparations" in Joseph P. Remington, *The Practice of Pharmacy*, 3rd ed. (Philadelphia: J. B. Lippincott, 1889), 1267–95.

9. John Uri Lloyd, "Polypharmacy," *EMJ* 47 (February 1887): 70–72.

10. Lloyd took care to explain and delineate the salient features of this legislation to his eclectic colleagues. Through his *Eclectic Medical Gleaner*, he printed a twenty-one-page pamphlet "The National Pure Food and Drug Act" in 1907, which explained the historical and practical necessity for the measure and detailed its provisions.

11. Haller, *Medical Protestants*, 143.

12. John King and Robert S. Newton, *The Eclectic Dispensatory of the United States of America* (Cincinnati: H. W. Derby, 1852), vi.

13. John King and John Uri Lloyd, *Supplement to the American Dispensatory* (Cincinnati: Wilstach, Baldwin, 1880), iv.

14. King and Lloyd, *Supplement*, iii.

15. Letter from Lloyd to Kremers, November 10, 1924, KRF, A2, file 16. It is impossible to verify all of Lloyd's assertions here, but Otto Juettner's *Daniel Drake and His Followers* does support Lloyd's outline of the career John F. Judge (1832–1891). He did indeed graduate from the EMI in 1854 and taught there until 1874 when he took course work at the Cincinnati College of Medicine and Surgery, an allopathic school. He taught chemistry for many years at the Cincinnati College of Pharmacy, and from 1879 to 1881 was on faculty at the Miami Medical College. Despite Lloyd's suggestions that relations between the EMI and Dr. Judge had deteriorated, Felter's 1902 *History of the Eclectic Medical Institute* included a highly complimentary sketch of J. F. Judge (pp. 125–26). As for the expulsion alluded to, there is no written record substantiating Lloyd's assertions.

16. *The Pharmacopeia of the United States of America,* 6th dec. rev. (New York: William Wood, 1882), xxxii–xxxiii.

17. See extant correspondence in LLM, coll. 1, box 12.

18. Anderson and Higby, *The Spirit of Voluntarism,* 131–33.

19. Sonnedecker, *History of Pharmacy,* 267.

20. "Book Notices," *EMJ* 40 (June 1880): 294–95.

21. See review in the *American Journal of Pharmacy* 52 (September 1880): 480.

22. *Druggists Circular* 25 (March 1881): 47.

23. *Druggists Circular* 25 (April 1881): 63.

24. Review in *EMJ* 41 (March 1881): 151–52.

25. See reviews in the *Druggist* 3 (April 1881): 101; and the *American Journal of Pharmacy* 53 (March 1881): 143.

26. Gregory J. Higby, "Publication of the National Formulary: A Turning Point for American Pharmacy," in *One Hundred Years of the National Formulary,* ed. Gregory J. Higby (Madison, WI: AIHP, 1989), 6–7.

27. Remington, *Practice of Pharmacy,* 1st ed., 1885, 283.

28. Higby, "Publication of the National Formulary," 8–9.

29. Letter from Lloyd to Kremers, May 21, 1920, KRF, A2, file 15.

30. See the *Pharmacopeia of the United States of America* (Boston: Wells and Lilly, 1820), 243, listing for "Tincture of Sulphuric Acid (formerly Elixir of Vitriol)." It was carried in subsequent editions through 1870 of *USP* V (p. 72) until it was finally dropped with a new Elixir Aurantii (Elixir of Orange) added to the *USP* VI (p. 92).

31. The 1905 *USP* VIII (pp. 123–24) listed only three elixirs, two of which (Elixir of Licorice and Elixir of Orange) were designed only as administration vehicles, and just one (Elixir of Iron, Quinine and Strychnine) consisted of any intended remedial value.

32. Review in the *American Journal of Pharmacy* 55 (August 1883): 430–31.

33. John Uri Lloyd, *Elixirs: Their History, Formulae, and Methods of Preparation* (Cincinnati: Robert Clarke, 1883), 3.

34. Higby, "Publication of the National Formulary," 11–15.

35. Despite its prominence in the 1st edition of the *NF,* the role of the elixir would diminish over time. See table II in Glenn Sonnedecker, "The Changing Character of the National Formulary (1890–1970)," in *One Hundred Years of the National Formulary,* 32.

36. Higby, "Publication of the National Formulary," 16.

37. *The National Formulary,* 6th ed. (Washington, DC: American Pharmaceutical Association, 1935), 485. Lloyd's contribution has been recognized in the *NF* ever since its first "Historical Introduction" in the 4th edition (1916), and it is still carried today: see the 1995 *NF* 18 (p. 2196).

38. See the "Prospectus" reprinted in John Uri Lloyd and Curtis Gates Lloyd, *Drugs and Medicines of North America,* Bulletin of the Lloyd Library of Botany, Pharmacy and Materia Medica 29 (Cincinnati: LLM, 1930), 1.

39. See reviews in the *Druggists Circular* 28 (May 1884): 79; the *Druggist* 6 (May 1884): 118; and the *American Journal of Pharmacy* 56 (June 1884): 346.

40. Edward Kremers, foreword to *Drugs and Medicines of North America,* by J. U. and C. G. Lloyd, n.p.

41. This conclusion concurs with that of Glenn Sonnedecker. See his "American Pharmaceutical Historiography I," 72–73.

42. Charles F. Millspaugh, *American Medicinal Plants*, 2 vols. (New York: Boericke & Tafel, 1887; Philadelphia: John C. Yorston, 1892).

43. For bibliographical details on all of these works, see appendix 4.

44. John Uri Lloyd, *Origin and History of All the Pharmacopeial Vegetable Drugs* (Cincinnati: Caxton Press, 1929), v–ix.

45. Sonnedecker, "American Pharmaceutical Historiography I," 73.

46. For details, see the annual announcements of the Eclectic Medical Institute and after 1910 the Eclectic Medical College Bulletins, LLM.

47. Rolla L. Thomas, "John Uri Lloyd—Teacher," *EMJ* 96 (May 1936): 197.

48. Letter from Charles L. Olsen to Harvey W. Felter, February 19, 1907, LLM, coll. 3, box 35, folder 1,035, p. 8. Olsen had graduated with the class of 1898 and was apparently replying to Felter's request for historical information on the faculty of the institute.

49. John Uri Lloyd, "Response" in Thomas, "John Uri Lloyd," 199–200.

50. Olsen, letter, LLM, coll. 3, box 35, folder 1,035, p. 2.

51. John Thomas Lloyd, "A Record of How John Uri Lloyd Lectured," LLM, coll. 3, box 23, folder 702.

52. Olsen, letter, LLM, coll. 3, box 35, folder 1,035, pp. 9–10.

53. Edward Kremers and George Urdang, *History of Pharmacy: A Guide and a Survey*, 2nd ed. (Philadelphia: Lippincott, 1951), 456.

8. Lloyd as Litterateur

1. A publisher's notice states that the first edition of 1,299 copies was sold in advance and that the so-called second edition (Robert Clarke's first printing) of a little more than 1,000 copies was sold within a week. They warned that the third printing "is being rapidly taken." See Notice, LLM, coll. 1, box 28, folder 401.

2. See, for example, Robert Reginald, *Science Fiction and Fantasy Literature: A Checklist, 1700–1974*, 2 vols. (Detroit: Gale Research, 1979) 1:324; and Peter Nicholls, ed. *The Science Fiction Encyclopedia* (Garden City, NY: Doubleday, 1979), 359–60.

3. John Uri Lloyd, *Etidorhpa, or The End of Earth*, 2nd ed. (Cincinnati: Robert Clarke, 1896; reprint, Santa Fe, NM: Sun Publishing, 1976). Beginning with the second edition, Lloyd excerpted reviews of *Etidorhpa* to be appended at the end of the novel. Despite the scarcity of the original author's edition, this later version is of more critical value. All references are to the second edition unless otherwise noted. It is important to note that these so-called editons really represent printings and that no textual changes were made until the eleventh and twelfth editions by the New York publishing house of Dodd, Mead. These later changes, however, are considered detrimental to the work as a whole. For details, see Laurel Black, "A Textual Study of *Editorhpa*," typescript, unpublished graduate paper, Miami University, 1989, LLM coll. 1, box 28, folder 405.

4. Charles Frederic Goss, *Cincinnati—The Queen City, 1788–1912*, (Chicago: S. J. Clarke, 1912), 3:740.

5. See reviews in the *Arena* 83 (October 1896): 855–57; and the *Arena* 77 (April 1896): 851–59.

6. Review of *Stringtown on the Pike* in the *Arena* 25 (March 1901): 340–42.

7. Review of *Stringtown on the Pike* in the *Dial* 29 (December 16, 1900): 498–99. It is interesting to note with regard to Lloyd's unusual title that dystopian author Sa-

muel Butler's *Erewhon* (1872), "nowhere" spelled backward, may have suggested his *Etidorhpa*.

8. Lloyd, *Etidorhpa*, 11.

9. Lloyd, *Etidorhpa*, 34.

10. Lloyd, *Etidorhpa*, 258.

11. Lloyd, *Etidorhpa*, 345–46.

12. Lloyd, *Etidorhpa*, 350–51.

13. See Edward H. Davidson, *Poe: A Critical Study* (Cambridge, MA: Harvard University Press, 1957), 156–80; and Michael Dirda, afterword to *A Journey to the Center of the Earth*, by Jules Verne (New York: New American Library, 1986), 289–90.

14. Quoted in Lloyd, *Etidorhpa*, 373.

15. For a brief history of hollow-earth theories, see Leslie Shepard, ed., *Encyclopedia of Occultism and Parapsychology*, 3rd ed. (Detroit: Gale Research, 1991), 1:770–71.

16. Although this pamphlet is not readily available, Cyrus Teed discusses his revelatory theories at length in *The Cellular Cosmogony, or, The Earth a Concave Sphere* (Estero, FL: Guiding Star Publishing, 1905; reprint, Philadelphia: Porcupine Press, 1975).

17. This is no small achievement. Although never attaining large-scale popularity itself, it has outlived all but two of the top ten national best-sellers of 1895. See Alice Payne Hackett, *70 Years of Best Sellers, 1895–1965* (New York: R. R. Bowker, 1967), 91.

18. The persistent devotion to this book by seers, mystics, and assorted self-styled visionaries is amazing. Several interesting anecdotes have been told of such visitors by the Lloyd Library librarian of some thirty years, Mrs. Simons. See Simons, *John Uri Lloyd*, 195.

19. See Kenneth M. Roemer, *The Obsolete Necessity: America in Utopian Writings, 1888–1900* (Kent, OH: Kent State University Press, 1976); and L. Thomas Williams, "Journeys to the Center of the Earth: Descent and Initiation in Selected Science Fiction," Ph.D. diss. (Bloomington: Indiana University, 1983).

20. L. Thomas Williams, "Journeys," 168–216.

21. Roemer, *Obsolete Necessity*, 24–199 passim.

22. Neil Wilgus, introduction to *Etidorhpa*, xi–xii.

23. For details on the utopian literary movement, see Arthur O. Lewis, "Utopia," *Dictionary of Literary Themes and Motifs* (New York: Greenwood Press, 1988), 2:1361–71.

24. Wilgus, introduction to *Etidorhpa*, xi–xii; and Roemer, *Obsolete Necessity*, 80–81.

25. John Uri Lloyd, "Back to the People. Down with Narcotics and Habit-Forming Drugs," *EMJ* 85 (May 1925): 5.

26. Terence McKenna, *The Archaic Revival* (San Francisco: Harper, 1991).

27. McKenna, *Archaic Revival*, 190.

28. Lloyd, *Etidorhpa*, 131.

29. McKenna, *Archaic Revival*, 193.

30. John Uri Lloyd, Wolfgang Ostwald, and Hans Erbring, "Physics and Pharmacy," *JAPhA* 23 (March 1934): 214.

31. See LLM, coll. 11, box 35, folder 1,035.

32. George B. Wood and Franklin Bache, *The Dispensatory of the United States of America*, 12th ed. (Philadelphia: J. B. Lippincott, 1866), 1561, states that Dr. B. W. Richardson first investigated the "remarkable narcotic and anaesthetic properties" of the puffball in 1853.

33. An original edition (undoubtedly read by the Lloyd brothers) is in the current Lloyd Library collection. See call number RC566 .C65.

34. See Edmund Ragland Badham, "Cultural Studies on the Mushroom *Psilocybe cubensis*," Ph.D. diss., City University of New York, 1983, 10–11.

35. John Uri Lloyd, "A Statement of Fact," LLM, coll. 1, box 28, folder 403. The witness's signature is that of William J. Miller, plant superintendent for the Lloyd Brothers firm.

36. Black, "Textual Study," LLM, coll. 1, box 28, folder 405.

37. Lloyd, "Statement," 3.

38. Lloyd, "Statement," 1.

39. Sonnedecker, "American Pharmaceutical Historiography I," 72.

40. John Uri Lloyd, *John King, M.D.*, Bulletin of the Lloyd Library of Botany, Pharmacy and Materia Medica 19 (Cincinnati: LLM, 1912), 12.

41. Published by Dodd, Mead, *Stringtown on the Pike: A Tale of Northernmost Kentucky* (New York, 1900) was simultaneously issued by Grosset & Dunlap and went through six printings until 1934. *Warwick of the Knobs: A Story of Stringtown County, Kentucky* (New York: Dodd, Mead, 1901) was also issued by the New York publishing houses of B. W. Dodge and Century that same year. Others in the series include *Red-Head* (New York: Dodd, Mead, 1903); *Scroggins* (New York: Dodd, Mead, 1904); *Felix Moses, the Beloved Jew of Stringtown on the Pike* (Cincinnati: Caxton Press, 1930); and *Our Willie: A Folklore Story of the Gunpowder Creek and Hills, Boone County, Kentucky* (Cincinnati: Caxton Press, 1934). For full details on all of the Stringtown novels, see Michael A. Flannery, "The Local Color of John Uri Lloyd: A Critical Survey of the Stringtown Novels," *Register of the Kentucky Historical Society* 91 (winter 1993): 24–50.

42. Grant C. Knight, *American Literature and Culture* (New York: Long & Smith, 1932), 343.

43. Merrill Maguire Skaggs, "Varieties of Local Color," in *The History of Southern Literature*, ed. Louis D. Rubin Jr. (Baton Rouge: Louisiana State University Press, 1985), 221.

44. Thomas D. Clark, *Kentucky: Land of Contrast* (New York: Harper & Row, 1968), ix.

45. These characteristics are offered and explained at length in Alice Hall Petry, *Local Color Fiction, 1870–1900*, Ph.D. diss., Brown University, 1979 (Ann Arbor: University Microfilms Inc., 1991), 65–204 passim. See also Eric Sundquist, "Realism and Regionalism," in *Columbia Literary History of the United States*, ed. Emory Elliott (New York: Columbia University Press, 1988), 501–24.

46. *St. Louis Daily Globe*, September 20, 1901, in LLM, coll. 1, box 20, scrapbook 3.

47. Lloyd and Lloyd, *Drugs and Medicines of North America*, 1:159.

48. Lloyd, *Stringtown*, 406.

49. Letter from Venable to Lloyd, January 7, 1901, LLM, coll. 1, box 13, folder 273.

50. *Cincinnati Times-Star*, January 12, 1901, reported that even with the library's large stock of the novel, supply could not keep pace with demand. LLM, coll. 1, box 20, scrapbook 3.

51. Reviewed in the *Arena* (March 1901): 340–42.

52. Reviewed in the *Dial* (December 16, 1900): 498–99; and the *Bookman* (December 1900): 352–53. The *Criterion* (January 1901): 9–10, offers the mixed blessings of such

literary pundits as William Dean Howells, F. Hopkins Smith, George Cary Eggleston, and Arthur Bartlett.

53. The proposed project spanned a number of years and is discussed in a series of letters between Lloyd and his publishers from July 6, 1915, until September 17, 1915. Picture rights were sold with the author receiving one-third of the projected proceeds. The plan lingered for a while but then collapsed when the film company went permanently out of business.

54. See LLM, coll. 1, box 2, folder 29.

55. Letter from James Knapp Reeve to Lloyd, January 25, 1898, LLM, coll. 1, box 31, folder 435.

56. *St. Louis Daily Globe*, September 20, 1901, LLM, coll. 1, box 20, scrapbook 3.

57. See John Wilson Townsend, *Kentucky in American Letters, 1784–1912* (Cedar Rapids, IA: Torch Press, 1913), 1:366–68.

58. Compare, for example, the general disdain for Burbridge's oath and his heavy-handed methods (*Warwick*, chapter 7) with the actual policy of retaliation meted out to Kentucky civilians as described in James A. Ramage, *Rebel Raider: The Life of John Hunt Morgan* (Lexington: University Press of Kentucky, 1986), 212–13. Here again, Lloyd was relying on personal experience and documentary evidence to depict actual events and attitudes. In a letter addressed to him headed "Florence, Ky., Aug. 10, 1864," his mother wrote, "I intend to keep my promise about writing you while things are so unsettled here. Mrs. Dulaney got home yesterday. Burbridge released her. Great indignation prevails everywhere in regard to her arrest." See LLM, coll. 1, box 6, folder 56.

59. Lloyd, *Warwick*, 71. Lloyd expressed his opinion openly in an angry reply to a Boston journalist's observations of the South during Reconstruction, LLM, coll. 1, box 40, folder 572. Although self-serving and obviously patronizing, Lloyd's opinion was quite common among the southern white intelligentsia.

60. See, for example, Ish Richey, *Kentucky Literature, 1784–1963* (Tompkinsville, KY: Monroe County Press, 1963), 48; and William S. Ward, *A Literary History of Kentucky* (Knoxville: University Press of Tennessee, 1988), 63.

61. *Warwick* ran serially in the *Bookman* from May through December 1901. Letter from Riley to Lloyd, December 13, 1901, coll. 1, box 11, folder 227.

62. John Uri Lloyd, "Grover Cleveland's opinion of 'Warwick of the Knobs,'" LLM, coll. 1, box 2, folder 21.

63. Lloyd, *Felix Moses*, 165–66.

64. Petry, *Local Color Fiction*, 176–77.

65. Lloyd, *Our Willie*, ix.

66. Ward, *Literary History*, 49.

67. Joseph V. Roney of Pharmacy Affairs, Hoechst-Roussel, made this discovery, and much to the author's gratitude, copied the photograph that is now among the holdings of the LLM.

68. There are four letters extant between Allen and Lloyd. One is undated; the others were written on May 20, 1895, October 11, 1895, and September 12, 1901. Originals in LLM, coll. 1, box 6, folder 67.

69. Knight, *James Lane Allen and the Genteel Tradition* (Chapel Hill: University of North Carolina Press, 1935), 101.

70. Knight, *James Lane Allen*, 71.

71. Letter from Allen to Lloyd, September 11, 1901, LLM, coll. 1, box 6, folder 67.

72. Knight, *James Lane Allen*, 119.

73. Knight, *James Lane Allen*, 70.

74. Letter from Allen to Lloyd, October 11, 1895, LLM, coll. 1, box 6, folder 67.

75. LLM, coll. 1, box 25, scrapbook 10.

9. THE BEST OF TIMES, THE WORST OF TIMES: FRIENDS, FOES, AND FAMILY

1. Letter from Emma Lloyd Nead to Curtis Gates, July 7, 1882, LLM, coll. 11, box 10, folder 209.

2. Schlereth, *Victorian America*, 276.

3. There is as yet no book-length study of Charles Rice. Until one is written, the best single source on Rice is H. George Wolfe, "Charles Rice (1841–1900), An Immigrant in Pharmacy," *American Journal of Pharmaceutical Education* 14 (April 1950): 285–305.

4. This incident is covered in Anderson and Higby, *The Spirit of Voluntarism*, 130–31. The original correspondence between Lloyd and Rice concerning the *USP* copyright issue, including the copy of a letter from Rice to John King, can be found in LLM, coll. 1, box 12, folders 257–58.

5. Letter from Rice to Lloyd, November 20, 1879, LLM, coll. 1, box 12, folder 257.

6. Letter from Rice to Lloyd, March 20, 1880, LLM, coll. 1, box 12, folder 257.

7. Letter from Rice to Lloyd, April 29, 1880, LLM, coll. 1, box 12, folder 257.

8. Anderson and Higby, *The Spirit of Voluntarism*, 128.

9. Letter from Rice to King, April 5, 1881, LLM, coll. 1, box 12, folder 258.

10. Letter from Rice to Lloyd, March 15, 1882, LLM, coll. 1, box 12, folder 259. Rice was of the opinion that Nelson Marvin Lloyd suffered from "senile gangrene" and stated that the physicians he consulted would not "venture a suggestion" as to treatment.

11. This book is still on the shelves of the Lloyd Library's rare book room. Lloyd thought so highly of the work that he reprinted it as Bulletin 3 of his Reproduction Series of the Lloyd Library in 1903.

12. Letter from Rice to Lloyd, May 19, 1884, LLM, coll. 1, box 12, folder 259.

13. Letter from Rice to Lloyd, november 12, 1884, LLM, coll. 1, box 12, folder 259.

14. Richard Hofstadter, *The American Political Tradition and the Men Who Made It* (New York: Vintage Books, 1948), 175–76.

15. See Hofstadter's quotation of Woodrow Wilson on Cleveland, 182.

16. Letter from Rice to Lloyd, April 10, 1901, LLM, coll. 1, box 12, folder 262.

17. See Wood and Bache's first mention of *Hydrastis canadensis* in the *USD*, 2nd ed. (Philadelphia: Grigg & Elliot, 1834), 1087.

18. Wood and Bache, *USD*, 14th ed. (Philadelphia: J. B. Lippincott, 1880), 488. See also John King and John Uri Lloyd's discussion of hydrastis in *The American Dispensatory*, rev. ed. (Cincinnati: Wilstach, Baldwin, 1886), 432–34.

19. Wood and Bache, *USD*, 14th ed., 487.

20. Edwin M. Hale, *New Remedies: Their Pathogenic Effects and Therapeutical Application in Homeopathic Practice* (Detroit: E. A. Lodge, 1864), 247–62.

21. Wood and Bache, *USD*, 14th ed., 488.

22. The Lloyds reprinted this from the serial version as J. U. and C. G. Lloyd, *Drugs and Medicines of North America*, Bulletin of the Lloyd Library of Botany, Pharmacy and Materia Medica 10 (Cincinnati: LLM, 1908). All subsequent references are to this edition.

23. Lloyd and Lloyd, *Drugs and Medicines*, 112.

24. Lloyd and Lloyd, *Drugs and Medicines*, 117.

25. *EMJ* 45 (August 1885): 399–400.

26. Wood and Bache, *USD*, 14th ed., 487. The irritant properties and dangers of hydrastis are reported in the literature today, even by those who believe the plant to have considerable therapeutic efficacy. Rosemary Gladstar writes, for example, that "goldenseal should only be used for a short period of time. Taken over an extended period, it builds up in the mucosa of the body, causing irritation and inflammation. Goldenseal should be used during pregnancy with caution," she adds. "Large doses stimulate the involuntary muscles of the uterus and may cause premature contractions." See *Herbal Healing for Women* (New York: Fireside, 1993), 29.

27. Samples of fliers and circulars are also available in LLM, coll. 6, box 6, folder 58; and LLM, coll. 6, box 10, folders 141–42. See also the pamphlet "presented with the compliments of Lloyd Brothers, Cincinnati, Ohio" titled "Hydrastis, the Favorite American Remedy . . . Lloyd's Hydrastis, the Standard Hydrastis Preparation." This curious sixteen-page promotional publication was directed at physicians and consisted of a mixture of history, excerpted articles, and advertisement copy extolling the superiority of Lloyd's Hydrastis. It was found tipped into the library's copy of the 1864 edition of Hale's *New Remedies* at the beginning of the section on hydrastis.

28. Letter from Rice to Lloyd, February 13, 1886, LLM, coll. 1, box 12, folder 260.

29. The objections of Lloyd's colleagues to product secrecy were rooted in medical precedent. English physician Thomas Percival was very clear on the secrecy of medicaments: "No physician or surgeon should dispense a secret *nostrum*, whether it be his invention, or exclusive property. For if it be of real efficacy, the concealment of it is inconsistent with beneficence and professional liberality. And if mystery alone give it value and importance, such craft implies either disgraceful ignorance, or fraudulent avarice." See his *Medical Ethics, or, A Code of Institutes and Precepts Adapted to the Professional Conduct of Physicians and Surgeons* (Manchester: S. Russell, 1803) 45. This principle was upheld in virtually every nineteenth-century American medical society's code of ethics. It was equally expressed in the first formal code of pharmaceutical ethics adopted by the Philadelphia College of Pharmacy in 1848 as a professional obligation "to discountenance the use of secret formulæ."

30. Letter from Remington to Lloyd, January 5, 1888, LLM, coll. 1, box 11, folder 223.

31. Lyman F. Kebler correctly notes that "the term 'Patent Medicine' applied to a medicine of secret composition is a misnomer" since "patent means open, not secret." He further points out that to consider all proprietary medicines fraudulent is also incorrect. The key resides in a combination of factors that include the target market for the product, the substantiation of claims for its efficacy (or lack thereof), and in independent analysis and assessment of the formula. See his "United States Patents Granted for Medicines During the Pioneer Years of the Patent Office," *J APhA* 24 (June 1935): 485.

32. See the constitution and by-laws in *Proceedings* 35 (1887): 653.

33. Letter from Remington to Lloyd, January 10, 1888, LLM, coll. 1, box 11, folder 223.

34. Letter from Lloyd to Remington, January 31, 1888, LLM, coll. 1, box 11, folder 223.

35. Joseph P. Remington, "Will Pharmacists Accept?" *American Journal of Pharmacy* 60 (February 1888): 67.

36. Letter from Lloyd to Ebert, February 11, 1888, KRF, A2, file 7.

37. Letter from Lloyd to Ebert, January 27, 1888, KRF, A2, file 7.

38. See postal inquiry letters from George E. Lorenz and John Riley, postmasters, September 13–14, 1888, LLM, coll. 1, box 11, folder 223.

39. *Bulletin of Pharmacy* 28 (January 1914): 3.

40. Quoted in Roland T. Lakey, "Frederick Stearns, Pharmacist," *J APhA*, Practical Pharmacy Edition 9 (August 1948): 487.

41. Liebenau, *Medical Science and Medical Industry*, 99.

42. Varro E. Tyler, *The Honest Herbal: A Sensible Guide to the Use of Herbs and Related Remedies*, 3rd ed. (New York: Pharmaceutical Products Press, 1993).

43. Andrew Weil, *Natural Medicine: A Comprehensive Manual for Wellness and Self-Care*, rev. ed. (Boston: Houghton Mifflin, 1995), 242. Advocacy of goldenseal in modern therapeutics can also be found in James A. Duke, *Handbook of Medicinal Herbs* (Boca Raton, FL: CRC Press, 1985), 238–39; *Lawrence Review of Natural Products* (May 1994), s.v. "Goldenseal"; Steven Foster, *Goldenseal*, Botanical Series 09 (Austin, TX: American Botanical Council, 1991); and David Hoffman and Diana DeLuca, *An Elder's Herbal: Natural Techniques for Promoting Health and Vitality* (Rochester, VT: Healing Arts Press, 1993), 225.

44. See "Public—No. 133," 17–18, LLM, coll. 1, box 18, folder 359.

45. Herbert B. Harding, "The History of Organization Among Manufacturers and Wholesale Dealers in Proprietary Articles," *American Druggist* 36 (March 26, 1900): 192.

46. John Uri Lloyd, "A Fragment of Unwritten History Concerning the Spanish War Tax, 1898," LLM, coll. 1, box 18, folder 361.

47. Lloyd, "Fragment of Unwritten History."

48. "Stamp Tax Muddle," *American Druggist* 36 (June 11, 1900): 416–17.

49. See Treasury Department Office of the Commissioner of Internal Revenue, "Opinion of the Attorney-General in Regard to the Taxability of Medicinal Preparations Under Schedule B, Act of June 13, 1898," *Department Circular 205; Internal Revenue 519*, December 22, 1898, p. 3, in LLM, coll. 1, box 18, folder 359.

50. Lloyd's materials on Grover Cleveland largely consist of newspaper clippings of their fishing trips. See LLM, coll. 1, box 20, scrapbook 9; and his separate book on Cleveland in coll. 1, box 20, scrapbook 1. There are personal letters between Lloyd and Cleveland that discuss Lloyd's Stringtown novels, but there is very little talk of politics.

51. See "Professor Lloyd Offered the Mayoralty," *Bulletin of Pharmacy* 25 (October 1911): 406.

52. Quoted in Glenn Sonnedecker, "Drug Standards Become Official," in *The Early Years of Federal Food and Drug Control*, ed. James Harvey Young (Madison, WI: AIHP, 1982), 28. See also James Harvey Young, *Pure Food: Securing the Federal Food and Drugs Act of 1906* (Princeton, NJ: Princeton University Press, 1989).

53. See John Uri Lloyd, "Physicians and the National Pure Food and Drug Act," *Eclectic Medical Gleaner* 3 (May 1907): 243–50; and Lloyd, "Eclectic Preparations and the National Pure Food and Drug Law," *Transactions of the National Eclectic Medical Association* 36 (1907–08): 45–51.

54. Lloyd, "Physicians," 246.

55. Lloyd, "Physicians," 250.

56. Lloyd, "Eclectic Preparations," 49.

57. Sonnedecker, "Drug Standards," 37.

58. "Lloyd's European Trip," *EMJ* 66 (March 1906): 159–60.

59. See, for example, Lloyd's report in the *Proceedings* 57 (1909): 648–49; Lloyd, "Opium Inspection in Smyrna," *Bulletin of Pharmacy* 21 (1907): 479; and Lloyd, "A Letter from the Orient: Mastic and Its Oriental Uses," *American Journal of Pharmacy* 89 (January 1917): 1–8.

60. Lloyd's experience with other cultures produced no epiphanic awakening like that described in the 1975 best-seller *The Tao of Physics* by theoretical physicist Fritjof Capra. This book, which attempts to blend and reconcile Eastern mysticism and Western scientific thought, has since been revised and is still in print as *The Tao of Physics: An Exploration of the Parallels Between Modern Physics and Eastern Mysticism*, 3rd ed. (Boston: Shambhala, 1991).

61. John Uri Lloyd, "Lloyd's Foreign Letter—No. 5," *EMJ* 66 (August 1906): 401.

62. The text of Lloyd's speech is available in George B. Griffenhagen, ed., *The Remington Lectures: A Century in American Pharmacy* (Washington, DC: American Pharmaceutical Association, 1994), 16–19.

10. THE LAST GREAT ECLECTIC

1. Lloyd, "Precipitates in Fluid Extracts," *Proceedings* 32 (1884): 418.

2. Lloyd, "Precipitates," *Proceedings* 32 (1884): 419.

3. See under "Capillarity" in *Chambers Science and Technology Dictionary* (Cambridge: Chambers, 1988), 131.

4. John Uri Lloyd and Sigmund Waldbott, *References to Capillarity*, Bulletin of the Lloyd Library of Botany, Pharmacy and Materia Medica 4 (Cincinnati: LLM, 1902).

5. For details, see entries for each scientist listed in the *DBS* and in the *Dictionary of the History of Science*, W. F. Bynum, E. J. Browne, and Roy Porter, eds. (Princeton, NJ: Princeton University Press, 1981), 51–52.

6. John Uri Lloyd, "Solvents in Pharmacy," *J APhA* 6 (November 1917): 944. These studies were continued in the *J APhA* 7 (February 1918): 137–49; and as part 1 of "Physics in Pharmacy," *J APhA* 11 (June 1922): 409–23.

7. See "Correspondence," *J APhA* 17 (August 1928): 820–21.

8. The first of these appeared as a continuation of Lloyd's part I of "Physics in Pharmacy" in John Uri Lloyd, Wolfgang Ostwald, and Walter Haller, "Physics in Pharmacy. Part II," *J APhA* 18 (September 1929): 862–75.

9. Lloyd, Ostwald, and Haller, "Physics in Pharmacy. Part II," 874.

10. See John Uri Lloyd, Wolfgang Ostwald, and Walter Haller, "A Study in Pharmacy," *J APhA* 19 (October 1930): 1076–89; and Lloyd, Ostwald, and Haller, "Physics in Pharmacy. Part III," *J APhA* 20 (February 1931): 95–110.

11. John Uri Lloyd, Wolfgang Ostwald, and Hans Erbring, "Physics in Pharmacy," *J APhA* 23 (March 1934): 214.

12. Jerome Alexander, ed., *Colloid Chemistry* (New York: Chemical Catalog, 1928), 2:931–934.

13. See *Remington's Practice of Pharmacy*, 8th ed. (Philadelphia: J. B. Lippincott, 1936), 202–10.

14. See the chapters on "Interfacial Phenomena" and "Colloidal Dispersions" in

Remington: The Science and Practice of Pharmacy, 19th ed., (Easton, PA: Mack Publishing, 1995), 1:241–77.

15. "Correspondence," *J APhA* 17 (August 1928): 820.

16. Kremers and Urdang, *History of Pharmacy*, 434.

17. Sonnedecker, *History of Pharmacy*, 51.

18. Sonnedecker, *History of Pharmacy*, 51–52.

19. See Robert A. Buerki, "Reception of the Germ Theory of Disease in The American Journal of Pharmacy," *Pharmacy in History* 13 (1971): 158–68.

20. The refusal of most eclectics to accept this paradigm of modern medicine is discussed at length in Haller, *Medical Protestants*, 190–92.

21. Quoted in Haller, *Medical Protestants*, 190–92.

22. John Uri Lloyd, "Nature's Products vs. Artificial," *EMJ* 48 (February 1888): 73–75.

23. John Uri Lloyd, "Medicine and Pharmacy in Revolt," *EMJ* 68 (July 1908): 357.

24. See, for example, John Uri Lloyd, "Back to the People," *EMJ* 70 (February 1910): 111–13.

25. John Parascandola, *The Development of American Pharmacy: John J. Abel and the Shaping of a Discipline* (Baltimore: Johns Hopkins University Press, 1992), 13. Parascandola gives an interesting account of the disciplinary shift in his chapter "From Materia Medica to Pharmacology," 1–21.

26. Letter from Lloyd to John Wilson Townsend, October 30, 1930, The Filson Club, Louisville, KY.

27. Lloyd, *Our Willie*, 316.

28. Haller, *Medical Protestants*, 230.

29. Haller, *Medical Protestants*, 245.

30. See the final letter dissolving the Eclectic Medical College from AMA secretary H. G. Weiskotten to Robert N. Gorman of the First National Bank, March 19, 1942, LLM, coll. 3, box 23, folder 692A.

31. After World War I, American manufacturers moved increasingly toward sophisticated research and development laboratory techniques. For details, see John P. Swann, "The Evolution of the American Pharmaceutical Industry," *Pharmacy in History* 37 (1995): 76–86.

32. See *John T. Lloyd Laboratories, Inc., John T. Lloyd and Albert N. Brown v. Lloyd Brothers Pharmacists, Inc. and S. B. Penick & Co.*, Sixth Circuit Court of Appeals, 1939. The permanent injunction was issued September 26, 1941. Despite this decree, John T. Lloyd Laboratories continued to produce a limited number of pharmaceuticals on a small scale. In 1950 the name became Lloyd and Dabney, Inc. John Thomas Lloyd died on May 25, 1970. Additional information is available in the John Thomas Lloyd papers, especially LLM, coll. 10, box 2, folder 27.

33. Gary L. Nelson, ed. *Pharmaceutical Company Histories* (Bismark, ND: Woodbine Publishing, 1983), 1:43.

34. Tyler, "Pharmaceutical Botany in the U.S.—Its Heyday, Decline, and Renascence," *Pharmacy in History* 38 (1996): 21.

35. Alex Berman, "The Impact of the Nineteenth Century Botanico-Medical Movement on American Pharmacy and Medicine," Ph.D. diss. (Madison: University of Wisconsin, 1954), 309.

36. While it is true that Lloyd could not possibly match the larger American firms

like Eli Lilly, Squibb, and Parke, Davis alone, an attitude less fixed on eclecticism might have gained Lloyd support from wider circles. As it was, Lloyd was giving away property and money ($50,000 in one year) to shore up a failing sectarian college. On these donations, see LLM, coll. 3, box 44, folder 1,128; and coll. 3, box 23, folder 700.

37. See, for example, Steven Foster, *Herbal Renaissance: Growing, Using, and Understanding Herbs in the Modern World* (Salt Lake City: Gibbs-Smith, 1993).

38. Mark Blumenthal, "Milestones in Pharmaceutical Botany Since 1960," *Pharmacy in History* 38 (1996): 25.

39. The full story of Lloyd's introduction to echinaceae is told in his "*Echinaceae Angustifolia*—History, Description and Adulteration," *Ellingwood's Therapeutist* 11 (March 1917): 101–4.

40. See John Uri Lloyd, *A Treatise on Echinaceae*, Drug Treatise 30 (Cincinnati: Lloyd Brothers, 1917); and Varro E. Tyler and Virginia M. Tyler, "John Uri Lloyd, Phr.M., Ph.D. 1849–1936," *Journal of Natural Products* 50 (January–February 1987): 2.

41. Compare Lloyd's *A Treatise on Crataegus*, Drug Treatise 29 (Cincinnati: Lloyd Brothers, 1917) with Max Wichtl, ed., *Herbal Drugs and Phytopharmaceuticals: A Handbook for Practice on a Scientific Basis*, trans. Norman Grainger Bisset (Boca Raton, FL: CRC Press, 1994), 166.

42. Compare Lloyd's *A Treatise on Scutellaria*, Drug Treatise 16 (Cincinnati: Lloyd Brothers, 1908) with Daniel B. Mowrey, *The Scientific Validation of Herbal Medicine* (New Canaan, CT: Keats Publishing, 1986), 163 passim.

43. Quoted in Murray Breeze, "John Uri Lloyd—Rebel," *EMJ* 96 (May 1936): 217.

Epilogue: Beyond the Persona, Beneath the Mask

1. Peter Gay, *The Naked Heart*, vol. 4 of *The Bourgeois Experience: Victoria to Freud* (New York: W. W. Norton, 1995), 3.

2. Gay, *The Naked Heart*, 149.

3. See, for example, Lloyd, "Fragments from an Autobiography," 303–11; and Lloyd, "A Pharmaceutical Apprenticeship," 1333.

4. John Uri Lloyd, "The Odium of Eclecticism," *Transactions of the Ohio Eclectic Medical Association for the Year 1898* (Cincinnati: Ohio Eclectic Medical Association, 1898), 110–12. Reprinted in the *EMJ* 59 (January 1899): 34–41; the *Chicago Medical Times* 32 (January 1899): 9–13; and again in the *EMJ* 76 (December 1916): 625–30.

5. Lloyd, "The Odium of Eclecticism," 113.

6. Lloyd, "The Odium of Eclecticism," 118–19.

7. Lloyd, "The Odium of Eclecticism," 122.

8. Lloyd to Kremers, November 5, 1898, KRF, A2, file 9.

9. Lloyd to Lyman, September 21, 1917, mss. AIHP 266, Lyman, box 10, folder 2, State Historical Society of Wisconsin Archives, Madison.

10. Lloyd declined an offer from Edward Kremers to "become a member of a progressive faculty" by pleading obligations that "prevent me at present now from a work of this kind." See Lloyd to Kremers, March 2, 1900, KRF, A2, file 10.

11. John Uri Lloyd, "Knowledge Versus Education," *Eclectic Medical Gleaner* 2 (January 1906): 72.

12. John Uri Lloyd, "The Professional Future," *EMJ* 67 (May 1907): 308–10.

13. John Uri Lloyd, "The Trend in Pharmacy," *The Western Druggist* 17 (August 1895): 325.

14. Lloyd to Kremers, September 13, 1895, KRF, A2, file 8.

15. Alex Berman, "A Striving For Scientific Respectability," *Bulletin of the History of Medicine* 30 (January–February 1956): 7–31.

16. Lloyd to Kremers, November 1, 1924, KRF, A2, file 16.

17. Kremers to Lloyd, November 5, 1924, KRF, A2, file 16.

18. Kremers to Lloyd, November 19, 1924, KRF, A2, file 16.

APPENDIX 2. A MODERN DRUG HOUSE

1. Letter from John Fearn, LLM, coll. 6, box 3, folder 1.

2. A green, fragrant topical analgesic and antiphlogistic agent devised by John Uri Lloyd in 1903. Its active ingredients included cayenne, tobacco, bloodroot, lobelia, and other natural products indigenous to North America. It was quite popular and was always one of Lloyd Brothers' top-selling preparations. Like all of Lloyd's products, it too was sold only to physicians and pharmacists.

APPENDIX 3. OSTWALD'S NOTE

1. Wolfgang Ostwald, *Kolloidchemische Beihefte*, bd. 8, hft. 6–7 (1916): 171–250.

2. "Liesegang (1896) discovered the peculiar rhythmic precipitations produced by diffusion in gels (Liesegang rings), an explanation of which, in terms of supersaturation was attempted by Ostwald." See J. R. Partington, *A History of Chemistry*, vol. 4 (New York: St. Martin's Press, 1964), 738.

Bibliographical Essay

PUBLISHED PRIMARY SOURCES

John Uri Lloyd's production of essays and editorials was prodigious. Most of his eclectic writings appeared in the *Eclectic Medical Journal* and in the *Eclectic Medical Gleaner*, which Lloyd published from 1905 to 1912 (see the "Publisher's Department" section in particular). Lloyd's most important scientific writings, however, as well as the record of his professional activities appear in the *Proceedings of the American Pharmaceutical Association [Proceedings]*, the *Journal of the American Pharmaceutical Association [J APhA]*, and the Bulletin of the Lloyd Library of Botany, Pharmacy and Materia Medica [Bulletin]. Published from 1900 through 1936, Lloyd's most significant contributions to the Lloyd Library Bulletins series include *References to Capillarity*, Bulletin 4 (Cincinnati: Lloyd Library, 1902), the most comprehensive annotated bibliography on the subject; *The Eclectic Alkaloids, Resins, Oleo-Resins and Concentrated Principles*, Bulletin 12 (Cincinnati: Lloyd Library, 1910), Lloyd's valuable historical discussion of the eclectic "concentration craze"; and, coauthored with his brother Curtis Gates Lloyd, *Drugs and Medicines of North America*, 3 vols., Bulletin 29–31 (Cincinnati: Lloyd Library, 1930–1931), an aborted serial project that includes thorough discussions of plants like hydrastis, lobelia, cimifuga, and certain selections from the *Ranunculaceae* family that the Lloyds felt were of importance in medicine. Further examinations into various medicinal plants can be found in Lloyd's thirty-one Drug Treatises published from 1904 to 1918 by Lloyd Brothers of Cincinnati.

A good source for information on Specific Medicines are the numerous editions of Lloyd Brothers' *Dose Book of Specific Medicines*. These books give an alphabetical listing of each product, accompanied by a facsimile label, brief description, specific use, and recommended dosage. Also useful is some of the preliminary matter such as the sections on "Concerning Specific Medicines," "A Glossary of Indicated Remedies and Disease Names and Definitions," "Maximum and Minimum Doses of Specific Medicines," "Synonyms and Common Names Used for Specific Medicines," and "Uses and Dosages of Specific Medicines."

Those interested in Lloyd's work in chemistry should see his "Solvents in Pharmacy," *J APhA* 6 (November 1917): 940–49, continued in *J APhA* 7 (1918): 137–49; his "Physics in Pharmacy," *J APhA* 11 (June 1922): 409–23, later continued by Lloyd, Wolfgang Ostwald, and Walter Haller under that same title in *J APhA* 18 (September 1929): 862–75 and *J APhA* 20 (February 1931): 95–110. Related works also include Lloyd, Ostwald, and Haller, "A Study in Pharmacy,"

J APhA 19 (October 1930): 1076–89, which continues Lloyd's discussion of "Solvents in Pharmacy" (1918); and Lloyd, Ostwald, and Hans Erbring's continuation of "Physics in Pharmacy" in *J APhA* 23 (March 1934): 214–21, and *J APhA* 23 (April 1934): 324–417. Much of Lloyd's early work in this area is summarized in his "Colloids in Pharmacy," in *Colloid Chemistry: Theoretical and Applied*, ed. Jerome Alexander, vol. 2 (New York: Chemical Catalog, 1928), 931–34. Also of interest in showing Lloyd's impact on the European foreign community of scholars is Wolfgang Ostwald's reprinting of Lloyd's work in his *Kolloidchemische Beihefte*, bd. 8, hft. 6–7 (1916): 171–250. All of John Uri Lloyd's book-length studies are cited in appendix 3.

Electicism and its relationship to Lloyd's professional life and his Specific Medicines is best understood by going to the original sources themselves. John Uri Lloyd was so intimately connected with this botanico-medical sect that eclecticism forms a collateral body of primary resource material relative to his career. In this regard, examination of the *Eclectic Medical Journal* is essential, for this publication more than any other offers a comprehensive window to the issues that animated the discussions of eclectic practitioners. For the eclectics' therapeutics and materia medica, see the various editions of John King's *American Dispensatory*; Finley Ellingwood's *Treatise on Therapeutics and Materia Medica* (Chicago: F. Ellingwood, 1898); Finley Ellingwood's *Eclectic Practice of Medicine*, 2 vols. (Chicago: Ellingwood Therapeutist Publishing, 1910); and Harvey Wickes Felter's *Eclectic Materia Medica, Pharmacology and Therapeutics* (Cincinnati: John K. Scudder, 1922). On the theory and practice behind Specific Medicines, see John Milton Scudder, *Specific Medication and Specific Medicines* (Cincinnati: Wilstach, Baldwin, 1870) and subsequent editions.

In addition to eclectic materials are the standard reference works in American pharmacy. In this regard, see editions of the following works contemporaneous with Lloyd: *The Pharmacopeia of the United States of America [USP]*, 6th decennial rev. (New York: William Wood, 1882); *The United States Dispensatory [USD]*, 14th–21st eds. (Philadelphia: J. B. Lippincott, 1880–1927); *The National Formulary of Unofficinal Preparations [NF]* (American Pharmaceutical Association, 1888); Edward Parrish, *A Treatise on Pharmacy*, 3rd ed. (Philadelphia: Blanchard & Lea, 1864); and Joseph P. Remington, *The Practice of Pharmacy* (Philadelphia: J. B. Lippincott, 1885).

Lloyd's first effort in fiction, *Etidorhpa, or The End of Earth* (Cincinnati: Robert Clarke, 1895) has had a long publishing history. Still in print today, the most prevalent edition is issued by Sun Publishing, a New Age publishing house in Santa Fe, New Mexico. Others are available, but to this author's knowledge only the Sun printing and the Simon & Schuster Pocket Books edition includes the 1976 introduction by Neil Wilgus (see chapter 8 for details). Lloyd's other ventures into fiction include *The Right Side of the Car* (Boston: Badger, 1897), a novella full of Victorian sentimentality; *Stringtown on the Pike* (New York:

Dodd, Mead, 1900), the first of the Stringtown novels and Lloyd's most famous work in that genre; and the rest of the series, *Warwick of the Knobs* (New York: Dodd, Mead, 1901); *Red-Head* (New York: Dodd, Mead, 1903); *Scroggins* (New York: Dodd, Mead, 1904); *Felix Moses, the Beloved Jew of Stringtown on the Pike* (Cincinnati: Caxton Press, 1930); and *Our Willie* (Cincinnati: John G. Kidd, 1934). In addition to his Stringtown novels, Lloyd also wrote a series of "Sam Hill" stories. In the same vein as his other local color fiction, these tales describe the antics of a fictional Kentucky character named Sam Hill. Originally written during the 1920s, they were primarily designed as raconteur pieces to be delivered to the Cincinnati Literary Club. Only a few were ever published during Lloyd's lifetime, but now most are available in print. See "The Sam Hill Stories of John Uri Lloyd," compiled and edited by Michael A. Flannery, *Northern Kentucky Heritage* (spring–summer 1994): 26–32; (fall–winter 1995): 27–36; and (spring–summer 1995): 24–34.

Besides Lloyd's own writings, primary material is also available in the local newspapers, which devoted considerable coverage to John Uri Lloyd's and Lloyd Brothers' activities. Although most of these are available in the Lloyd Library scrapbooks, the researcher will find the Public Library of Cincinnati and Hamilton County's computerized NEWSDEX database an extremely handy source for area newspaper articles published since 1900. The Lloyds are well represented in this index.

Unpublished Primary Sources

The main repository of manuscripts and correspondence related to John Uri Lloyd are located at the Lloyd Library and Museum, 917 Plum Street, Cincinnati, Ohio 45202. Researchers interested in accessing this sizable body of material should first consult my article "The Life and Times of John Uri Lloyd: A View from the Archives of the Lloyd Library," *Pharmacy in History* 38 (1996): 107–20. This article gives an overview of the collection as it relates to Lloyd, plus an index of pharmacy-related archives at the library. Besides the Lloyd Library, the Kremers Reference Files, F. B. Power Pharmaceutical Library, University of Wisconsin, Madison, Wisconsin 53706, contains an extremely valuable body of material. The Lloyd materials in this collection comprise thirty-five files in three drawers marked A2. Among the more important items is the extensive correspondence between Lloyd and Edward Kremers, the heart of which can be found in the files numbered 6 through 21. These letters reveal interesting details concerning Lloyd's professional and personal life not otherwise available. In addition to Lloyd's correspondence, there are four files on the Lloyd Library. Those wishing access to this collection should contact the American Institute of the History of Pharmacy [AIHP], 425 North Charter Street, Madison, Wisconsin 53706. Also in Madison are the archives of the State Historical Society of Wisconsin. Among the more pertinent materials in this collection are holdings for Edward Kremers and Rufus A. Lyman, which contain Lloyd correspondence.

The only other body of material warranting mention is the correspondence between Lloyd, Grover Cleveland, and F. F. C. Preston. For a listing, see the *Index to the Grover Cleveland Papers* (Washington, DC: Library of Congress, 1965), 195.

SECONDARY SOURCES

Biographies

The most extensive treatment of John Uri Lloyd has been Corinne Miller Simons, *John Uri Lloyd, His Life and His Works, 1849–1936* (Cincinnati: C. M. Simons, 1972). Although it is a lengthy biography of more than three hundred pages, the book is unreferenced and unanalytical. Researchers should consult the Simons book with caution; errors abound and many statements are unverified.

Briefer but more informative biographical discussions can be found in the journal literature. One of the most important is the John Uri Lloyd memorial issue of the *Eclectic Medical Journal* 96 (May 1936). Included are reminiscences of Lloyd's colleagues and friends and various reprintings of his autobiographical addresses. Discussion of Lloyd's scientific career has been well summarized by John Parascandola; see under Lloyd, John Uri, in the *Dictionary of Scientific Biography*, ed. Charles Coulston Gillispie (New York: Charles Scribner's, 1973). Some general biographies include Roy Bird Cook, "John Uri Lloyd: Pharmacist, Philosopher, Author, Man," *JAPhA*, Practical Pharmacy Edition 10 (September 1949): 538–44; George D. Beal, "Lloyds of Cincinnati," *American Journal of Pharmaceutical Education* 23 (spring 1959): 202–6; Varro E. Tyler and Virginia M. Tyler, "John Uri Lloyd, Phr.M., Ph.D., 1849–1936," *Journal of Natural Products* 50 (January–February 1987): 1–8; and Michael A. Flannery, "John Uri Lloyd: The Life and Legacy of an Illustrious Heretic," *Queen City Heritage* 50 (fall 1992): 2–14.

Significant in demonstrating Lloyd's stature in the European community is his inclusion in Swiss pharmacist Burkhard Reber's *Gallerie hervorragender Therapeutiker und Pharmakognosten der Gegenwart* (Geneva: Paul Dubois, 1894). A typescript translation Reber's *Gallery of Prominent Therapists and Pharmacognosists of the Present* is available at the Lloyd Library.

The Lloyd Library and Museum

Information on the Lloyd Library is available in Caswell A. Mayo, *The Lloyd Library and Its Makers: An Historical Sketch*, Bulletin of the Lloyd Library of Botany, Pharmacy and Materia Medica 28 (Cincinnati: Lloyd Library, 1928); Corinne Miller Simons, "Lloyd Library and Museum: A History of Its Resources," *Special Libraries* 34 (December 1943): 481–86; Simons, "Lloyd Library," *Cincinnati Journal of Medicine* 58 (1972): 185–88; and Michael A. Flannery, "Ar chives of Phytomedicine at the Lloyd Library and Museum," *HerbalGram* 36 (1996): 42–48.

The growth of the Lloyd Library is best understood within the context of larger developments in research and research libraries. Three excellent studies are Samuel Rothstein, "The Context for Reference Service: The Rise of Research and Research Libraries, 1850–1900," Kenneth Brough, "The Heart of the University," and David Mearns, "The Library of Congress Under Putnam," in Michael H. Harris, ed., *Reader in American Library History* (Washington, DC: NCR Microcard, 1971).

Literary Criticism

On Lloyd's literary efforts, readers should see discussions in John Wilson Townsend, *Kentucky in American Letters, 1782–1912*, vol. 1 (Cedar Rapids, IA: Torch Press, 1913), 364–68; Eunice Bonow Bardell, "The Novels of the American Pharmacist, John Uri Lloyd," *Pharmacy in History* 29 (1987): 177–80; William S. Ward, *A Literary History of Kentucky* (Knoxville: University of Tennessee Press, 1988), 62–64; and Michael A. Flannery, "The Local Color of John Uri Lloyd: A Critical Survey of the Stringtown Novels," *The Register of the Kentucky Historical Society* 91 (winter 1993): 24–50.

More general sources on the local color literary movement include Grant C. Knight, *American Literature and Culture* (New York: Ray Long & Richard R. Smith, 1932), 343–357; Ludwig Lewisohn, *The Story of American Literature* (New York: Modern Library, 1939), 281–296; Eric J. Sundquist, "Realism and Regionalism," in *Columbia Literary History of the United States*, ed. Emory Elliott (New York: Columbia University Press, 1988), 501–24; the informative introduction and "Linguistic Note" by editors Walter Blair and Raven I. McDavid Jr. in *The Mirth of a Nation: America's Great Dialect Humor* (Minneapolis: University of Minnesota Press, 1983); and Alice Hall Petry's *Local Color Fiction, 1870–1900*, Ph.D. diss., Brown University, 1979 (Ann Arbor: University Microfilms Inc., 1991). Researchers will find Petry's dissertation the most thorough and comprehensive study of this interesting literary genre.

Pharmacy and Chemistry

The most authoritative single source on the history of pharmacy in English is *Kremers and Urdang's History of Pharmacy*, revised by Glenn Sonnedecker, 4th ed. (1976; Madison, WI: AIHP, 1986), but additional material on Lloyd and other aspects of the discipline related to Lloyd can be found in the earlier edition of that work by Edward Kremers and George Urdang, *History of Pharmacy: A Guide and a Survey*, 2nd ed. (Philadelphia: J. B. Lippincott, 1951). Also very helpful is David L. Cowen and William H. Helfand's *Pharmacy: An Illustrated History* (New York: Harry N. Abrams, 1990). These three basic sources cover the broad sweep of pharmaceutical history and are essential to placing Lloyd within the larger context of the discipline's development.

More specific but equally valuable in tracing the dramatic transformations in pharmacy during Lloyd's lifetime are the following: George Urdang, *Pharmacy's Part in Society* (Madison, WI: AIHP, 1946); Robert A. Buerki, "Reception of the Germ Theory of Disease in the American Journal of Pharmacy," *Pharmacy in History* 13 (1971): 158–68; Gregory J. Higby, "Professionalism and the Nineteenth-Century American Pharmacist," *Pharmacy in History* 28 (1986): 115–34; John P. Swann, "Biomedical Research and Government Support: The Case of Drug Development," *Pharmacy in History* 31 (1989): 103–16; Jonathan Liebenau, *Medical Science and Medical Industry: The Formation of the American Pharmaceutical Industry* (Baltimore: Johns Hopkins University Press, 1987); *Pill Peddlers: Essays on the History of the Pharmaceutical Industry*, ed. Gregory J. Higby and Elaine C. Stroud (Madison, WI: AIHP, 1990); John P. Swann, "The History of Pharmacy and Estates of Pharmacy: Institutional Frameworks for Drug Research in America," *Pharmacy in History* 32 (1990): 3–11; John Parascandola, "The Emergence of Pharmaceutical Science," *Pharmacy in History* 37 (1995): 68–75; and in that same issue, John P. Swann, "The Evolution of the American Pharmaceutical Industry," 76–86. An interesting discussion of the final sale of Lloyd Brothers of Cincinnati to Hoechst can be found in *Pharmaceutical Company Histories*, ed. Gary L. Nelson, vol. 1 (Bismarck, ND: Woodbine Publishing, 1983). Especially informative for his discussion of the shift from the empirical examination of crude drug products toward the systematic laboratory analysis characterized by the new specialty of pharmacology is John Parascandola's *Development of American Pharmacology: John J. Abel and the Shaping of a Discipline* (Baltimore: Johns Hopkins University Press, 1992).

On the development of *The National Formulary* and *The United States Pharmacopeia*, see the essays collected in *One Hundred Years of the National Formulary: A Symposium*, ed. Gregory J. Higby (Madison, WI: AIHP, 1989); and Lee Anderson and Gregory J. Higby, *The Spirit of Voluntarism: A Legacy of Commitment and Contribution: The United States Pharmacopeia, 1820–1995* (Rockville, MD: USP Convention, 1995).

Background and discussion on the Pure Food and Drug Act of 1906 is available in *Federal Food, Drug and Cosmetic Law Administrative Reports, 1907–1949* (Chicago: Commerce Clearing House, 1951). This is a compilation of material that includes the important reports of U.S. Department of Agriculture Bureau of Chemistry Chief Harvey W. Wiley (1844–1930). This book can be considered an important primary source for information related to the Pure Food and Drug Act of 1906, but because Lloyd had no direct involvement in its development, it has been included under secondary sources. Wiley provides an interesting, albeit partisan, account of opposition to the act in his *History of a Crime Against the Food Law: The Amazing Story of the National Food and Drugs Law Intended to Protect the Health of the People Perverted to Protect Adulteration of Foods and Drugs* (Washington, DC: H. W. Wiley, 1929). Other historical data on the Act can be found in Stephen Wilson, *Food and Drug Regulation* (Washington,

DC: American Council on Public Affairs, 1942); and *The Early Years of Federal Food and Drug Control* (Madison, WI: AIHP, 1982).

Finally, Lloyd's contributions to the history of pharmacy are candidly assessed in Glenn Sonnedecker's "American Pharmaceutical Historiography I," in *Pharmaceutical Historiography: Proceedings of a Colloquium Sponsored by the American Institute of the History of Pharmacy on the Occasion of the Institute's 25th Anniversary, Madison, Wisconsin, January 22–23, 1966,* ed. Alex Berman (Madison: AIHP, 1967), 72–74.

In the field of chemistry, several sources can help set the context of Lloyd's work. The classic treatment can be found in J. R. Partington, *A Short History of Chemistry,* 3rd ed. (New York: St. Martin's Press, 1957; New York: Dover Publications, 1989). Also helpful is William A. Tilden, *A Short History of the Progress of Chemistry in Our Own Times* (New York: Longmans, Green, 1899); and W. H. Brock, *The Norton History of Chemistry* (New York: W. W. Norton, 1993). For a discussion of colloidal chemistry during Lloyd's active research in that specialty see, Wolfgang Ostwald, *An Introduction to Theoretical and Applied Colloid Chemistry,* trans. Martin H. Fischer (New York: John Wiley, 1917). Ostwald specifically mentions Lloyd's contributions to the field.

Eclecticism

Anyone interested in eclecticism in American medicine must also understand the context of the botanico-medical movement in this country. Despite its age, the most thorough treatment of the subject remains Alex Berman's "Impact of the Nineteenth Century Botanico-Medical Movement on American Pharmacy and Medicine," Ph.D. diss. (Madison: University of Wisconsin, 1954). Various aspects of Berman's treatment of this sectarian phenomenon have been published as "The Heroic Approach in 19th Century Therapeutics," *Bulletin of the American Society of Hospital Pharmacists* (September–October 1954): 321–27; "A Striving for Scientific Respectability: Some American Botanics and the Nineteenth-Century Plant Materia Medica," *Bulletin of the History of Medicine* 30 (January–February 1956): 7–31; and "The Botanic Pracitioners of 19th-Century America," *American Professional Pharmacist* (October 1957): 866–70, 911–12. Additional coverage is given in Madge E. Pickard and R. Carlyle Buley, *The Midwest Pioneer: His Ills, His Cures, and Doctors* (New York: Henry Schuman, 1946); and in parts III and IV of William G. Rothstein's *American Physicians in the Nineteenth Century: From Sects to Science* (Baltimore: Johns Hopkins University Press, 1972).

The starting point for any research into American eclecticism are two classic sources: one by Alexander Wilder, *History of Medicine* (Augusta, ME: Maine Farmer Publishing, 1904); and another by Harvey Wickes Felter, *History of the Eclectic Medical Institute* (Cincinnati: Alumnal Association, 1902). The Felter book, in particular, contains valuable biographical sketches of institute faculty. For an even earlier treatment of eclecticism, see G. W. L. Bickley's "History of the Eclectic Medical Institute," *EMJ* 16 (January 1857): 9–15; (February 1857): 57–64; (March 1857): 105–12; and (April 1857): 153–156.

The most comprehensive and objective account of eclecticism is by John S. Haller Jr., *Medical Protestants: The Eclectics in American Medicine, 1825–1939* (Carbondale: Southern Illinois University Press, 1994). Other modern treatments of these medical sectarians are available in Ralph Taylor, "The Formation of the Eclectic School in Cincinnati," *Ohio State Archaeological and Historical Quarterly* 51 (October–December 1942): 279–88; Alex Berman, "Wooster Beach and the Early Eclectics," *University of Michigan Medical Bulletin* 24 (July 1958): 277–86; Ronald L. Numbers, "The Making of an Eclectic Physician: Joseph M. McElhinney and the Eclectic Medical Institute of Cincinnati," *Bulletin of the History of Medicine* 47 (March–April 1973): 155–66; and Alex Berman, "The Eclectic 'Concentrations' and American Pharmacy (1847–1861)," *Pharmacy in History* 22 (1980): 91–103.

Also, Francis Brinker and Katherine Rosson with Eclectic Medical Publications have begun reprinting original eclectic writings and informing them with current naturopathic commentaries and analysis in their serial, *The Eclectic Medical Journals*, first issued in 1995.

Medicine

General histories of medicine in the United States abound, but most helpful in this study were those that focused particularly upon the paradigmatic transformations in nineteenth-century medical practice and its impact upon therapeutics. In that regard, two of the most helpful books were Lester S. King's *Transformations in American Medicine from Benjamin Rush to William Osler* (Baltimore: Johns Hopkins University Press, 1991); and W. F. Bynum's *Science and the Practice of Medicine in the Nineteenth Century* (New York: Cambridge University Press, 1994).

For general discussions of the development of sectarian medical practice in America, see the essays collected in *Medicine Without Doctors: Home Health Care in American History*, ed. Guenter B. Risse and Ronald L. Numbers (New York: Science History Publications, 1977); and *Other Healers: Unorthodox Medicine in America*, ed. Norman Gevitz (Baltimore: Johns Hopkins University Press, 1988).

For the local medical scene in Cincinnati during Lloyd's lifetime, see the classic by Otto Juettner, *Daniel Drake and His Followers: Historical and Biographical Sketches* (Cincinnati: Harvey Publishing, 1909). Also of use is Reginald C. McGrane, *The Cincinnati Doctor's Forum* (Cincinnati: Academy of Medicine, 1957), a centennial history of the Academy of Medicine of Cincinnati.

Lloyd's contributions to medical botany and phytochemistry have already been documented. It is helpful and important, however, to place his work within the context of the general history of natural products. The best current sources are the published presentations of a symposium, Milestones of Pharmaceutical

Botany, sponsored by the American Institute of the History of Pharmacy at its annual meeting in Orlando, Florida, March 20, 1995. Ara Der Mardersonian's "Milestones of Pharmaceutical Botany: Pre-history to 1900"; Varro E. Tyler's "Pharmaceutical Botany in the U.S.—1900–1962"; and Mark Blumenthal's "Milestones in Pharmaceutical Botany Since 1960" is an excellent history of the vicissitudes of the vegetable kingdom in the healing arts by three well-known authorities on the subject. They all appear in *Pharmacy in History* 38.1 (1996). Another interesting treatment of natural products in history is John Mann's *Murder, Magic, and Medicine* (New York: Oxford University Press, 1994). For general sources on botanical medicine, see Richard Le Strange, *A History of Herbal Plants* (New York: Arco Publishing, 1977); Barbara Griggs, *Green Pharmacy: The History and Evolution of Western Herbal Medicine* (Rochester, VT: Healing Arts Press, 1981); Mark Evans, *Herbal Plants: History and Uses* (London: Studio Editions, 1991); and David J. Bellamy, *World Medicine: Plants, Patients, and People* (Cambridge, MA: Oxford University Press, 1992).

For current uses of medicinal plants, see the alphabetical listing of individual plant names in *The Lawrence Review of Natural Products*; Mark Blumenthal et al., eds., *German Commission E Monographs*, trans. S. Klein and R. S. Rister (Austin, TX: American Botanical Council, in press); Max Wichtl, ed., *Herbal Drugs and Phytopharmaceuticals: A Handbook for Practice on a Scientific Basis*, trans. Norman Grainger Bisset (Boca Raton, FL: CRC Press, 1994); and James E. Robbers, Marilyn K. Speedie, and Varro E. Tyler, *Pharmacognosy and Pharmacobiotechnology* (Baltimore: Williams & Wilkins, 1996). Other informative sources on current phytomedicines include James A. Duke, *Handbook of Medicinal Herbs* (Boca Raton, FL: CRC Press, 1985); Daniel B. Mowrey, *The Scientific Validation of Herbal Medicine* (New Canaan, CT: Keats Publishing, 1986); Ara Der Marderosian and Lawrence Liberti, *Natural Product Medicine: A Scientific Guide to Foods, Drugs, Cosmetics* (Philadelphia: George F. Stickley, 1988); and Varro E. Tyler, *The Honest Herbal: A Sensible Guide to the Use of Herbs and Related Remedies*, 3rd ed. (New York: Pharmaceutical Products Press, 1993).

Social and Political Milieu

Because Lloyd's adult life was spent in Cincinnati, an understanding of social, economic, and political development in this nineteenth-century river community is essential. A good starting point is Daniel Hurley's *Cincinnati, The Queen City* (Cincinnati: Cincinnati Historical Society, 1982). The WPA Guide series *Cincinnati: A Guide to the Queen City and Its Neighbors* (1943; Cincinnati: Cincinnati Historical Society, 1987), which includes Lloyd Brothers Pharmacists, Inc. (300 West Court Street), the Lloyd Library (309 West Court Street), and both John Uri Lloyd homes (3901 Clifton Avenue, and Harris and Lloyd Avenues in Norwood) as points of interest on its walking tours, also contains valuable material. Another interesting overview of the Queen City is provided by Alvin F. Harlow, *The Serene Cincinnatians* (New York: E. P. Dutton, 1950). An important historical source covering the city during Lloyd's youth is Henry A. Ford and Kate B. Ford, *History of Cincinnati, Ohio, with Illustrations and Biographical Sketches* (1881; Cincinnati: Ohio Book Store, 1987). The Fords also include some informative data on nineteenth-century medical practice, hospitals, and medical schools in the city. One final but very useful source comes from the pen of German traveler Friedrich Ratzel, who toured the United States from August 1873 through October 1874, taking meticulous notes along the way. His observations of the bustling river community of Cincinnati captures in vivid detail the city as Lloyd would have known it as a young man. See Ratzel's *Sketches of Urban and Cultural Life in North America*, trans. and ed. Stewart A. Stehlin (New Brunswick, NJ: Rutgers University Press, 1988).

Lloyd's own political philosophy and social views were in large part shaped by his experiences as a boy in Kentucky. This lies at the heart of his southern sympathies and his view that Kentucky had a special historical bond with the vanquished South. Nowhere is this idea given greater expression than in E. Merton Coulter's *Civil War and Readjustment in Kentucky* (Chapel Hill: University of North Carolina Press, 1926). Coulter, on faculty at the University of Georgia, scorned Reconstruction and argued that Kentucky engaged in a justifiable intellectual secession from the Union *after* the Civil War. In some limited but important senses, Lloyd echoed Coulter's thesis. For a description of Kentucky during Lloyd's boyhood years, see Susan S. Kissel and Margery T. Rouse, eds., *The Story of the Pewter Basin and Other Occasional Writings Collected in Southern Ohio and Northern Kentucky* (Bloomington, IN: T.I.S. Publications, 1981); and Lowell H. Harrison, *The Civil War in Kentucky* (Lexington: University Press of Kentucky, 1975).

For the social and intellectual life of the period, see the collection of essays in Daniel Walker Howe, ed., *Victorian America* (Philadelphia: University of Pennsylvania Press, 1976); Robert H. Wiebe, *The Search for Order, 1877–1920* (New York: Hill & Wang, 1967); Daniel E. Sutherland, *The Expansion of Everyday Life, 1860–1876* (New York: Harper & Row, 1989); and Thomas J. Schlereth, *Victorian America: Transformations in Everyday Life, 1876–1915* (New York: HarperCollins, 1991). Most helpful in delineating Lloyd's character within the context of his times is Peter Gay's *Naked Heart*, vol. 4 of *The Bourgeois Experience: Victoria to Freud* (New York: W. W. Norton, 1995).

Lloyd's pharmaceutical manufacturing and his professional concerns must be placed within the general business and political environment of the last half of the nineteenth century. Two helpful studies in this area are Alfred L. Thimm's *Business Ideologies in the Reform-Progressive Era, 1880–1914* (Tuscaloosa: University of Alabama Press, 1976); and Alan Trachtenberg's *Incorporation of America: Culture and Society in the Gilded Age* (New York: Hill & Wang, 1982). Richard Hofstadter analyzes the politics of corruption, the Grover Cleveland administration, and the personalities of the Progressive era in his *American Political Tradition and the Men Who Made It* (New York: Vintage Books, 1948).

Index

MICHAEL A. FLANNERY, the director of the Lloyd Library and Museum, Cincinnati, Ohio, received his B.A. from Northern Kentucky University, his M.L.S. from the University of Kentucky, and his M.A. in history from California State University at Dominguez Hills. In addition to his directorship, he holds appointments on the adjunct faculty of Northern Kentucky University's Department of History and the University of Cincinnati's College of Pharmacy. His essays on various aspects of pharmaceutical history have appeared in *HerbalGram*, the *Herbarist*, the *Register of the Kentucky Historical Society*, and *Pharmacy in History*. He received the 1995 Fischelis grant from the American Institute of the History of Pharmacy to pursue the present study on John Uri Lloyd.